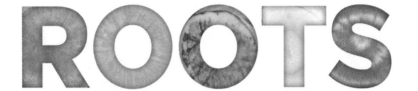

ROASTED ROOT VEGETABLES (page 136)

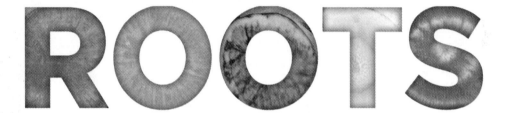 ROOTS

The Complete Guide to the
UNDERGROUND SUPERFOOD

STEPHANIE PEDERSEN

STERLING
New York

To Richard, Leif, Anders, and Axel. I love you!

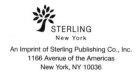

STERLING
New York

An Imprint of Sterling Publishing Co., Inc.
1166 Avenue of the Americas
New York, NY 10036

Text © 2017 by Stephanie Pedersen
Cover and interior photography © 2017 by Sterling Publishing Co, Inc., except where noted in the credits on page 171.

ISBN 978-1-4549-2142-4

Library of Congress Cataloging-in-Publication Data

Names: Pedersen, Stephanie, author.
Title: Roots : the complete guide to the underground superfood / Stephanie
   Pedersen.
Description: New York : Sterling, 2017. | Series: Superfoods for life
Identifiers: LCCN 2016045534 | ISBN 9781454921424 (paperback)
Subjects: LCSH: Cooking (Vegetables) | Root crops. | BISAC: COOKING / Health
   & Healing / General. | COOKING / Specific Ingredients / Natural Foods.
   HEALTH & FITNESS / Nutrition. | LCGFT: Cookbooks.
Classification: LCC TX801 .P39 2017 | DDC 641.6/5--dc23 LC record available at https://lccn.loc.gov/2016045534

Distributed in Canada by Sterling Publishing Co., Inc.
^c/o Canadian Manda Group, 664 Annette Street
Toronto, Ontario, Canada M6S 2C8
Distributed in the United Kingdom by GMC Distribution Services
Castle Place, 166 High Street, Lewes, East Sussex, England BN7 1XU
Distributed in Australia by NewSouth Books
45 Beach Street, Coogee, NSW 2034, Australia

For information about custom editions, special sales, and premium and corporate purchases, please contact
Sterling Special Sales at 800-805-5489 or specialsales@sterlingpublishing.com.

Manufactured in Canada

2 4 6 8 10 9 7 5 3 1

www.sterlingpublishing.com

CONTENTS

Introduction vi

CHAPTER 1: All About the Roots 1

CHAPTER 2: Drinks 41

CHAPTER 3: Breakfast 51

CHAPTER 4: Lunch 77

CHAPTER 5: Snacks 99

CHAPTER 6: Condiments 107

CHAPTER 7: Dinner 123

CHAPTER 8: Desserts 145

CHAPTER 9: Beauty 161

CHAPTER 10: Frequently Asked Questions 167

Photo Credits 171

Resources 172

Acknowledgments 174

About the Author 175

Index 176

What I say is that, if a fellow really likes potatoes, he must be a pretty decent sort of fellow.
—A. A. Milne

Solid, dependable, and comforting, root vegetables have sustained generations of people around the world: Think about the parsnip- and carrot-laden stews of northern Europe, the turnips and greens of the American South, the groundnut and sweet potato soup of Africa, the burdock-accented broths of China and Japan, the roasted rutabaga and pureed celeriac of Scandinavia, and more.

The humble root continues to be celebrated for its part in our culinary past. But there's more to a root veggie than its place in history. Take the potato, for instance—one of the world's most popular root veggies. According to the USDA, potatoes are the most frequently eaten vegetable in the United States, where 55 pounds of frozen potatoes, 42 pounds of fresh potatoes, 17 pounds of potato chips, and 14 pounds of dehydrated potato products are consumed on average, per capita per year. According to the Produce for Better Health Foundation, carrots are the fifth most consumed vegetable in the U.S., while sweet potatoes are the eleventh most popular vegetable in the root hit parade.

For many of us, root veggies are a reminder of childhood—foods we grew up eating. Microgreens and broccoli rabe and bok choy were—alas—completely unknown during my own childhood, but there were plenty of carrots, and radishes, and potatoes. These easy-to-grow, economical, long-storing vegetables played a big role in my childhood. Most of the meals my mother made consisted of a casserole, with a side of cooked veggies, such as carrots, or a salad, plus mashed potatoes or pickled beets. Sometimes there was a plate of radishes, served with a little dish of salt, or a pot roast accessorized with roasted potatoes. When I was at my grandmother's home, it was a turkey, a goose, or pork roasted in a pan, with various roots and a side of boiled red potatoes that were dusted with chopped parsley. For treats we enjoyed the ever-popular, cassava-based tapioca pudding.

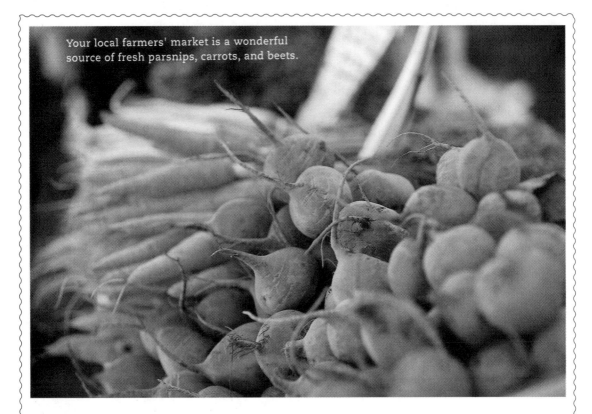

Your local farmers' market is a wonderful source of fresh parsnips, carrots, and beets.

My sister and I would complain about its bumpy, "frog eye" texture, but we did love its sweet, milky flavor.

For us, roots were just another part of a meal—and they were a part of our food supply. I grew up in a family that always kept a year's supply of food, because of our religious beliefs. This meant that a lot of potatoes (fresh and dried) and carrots (fresh and canned) and beets (pickled) were tucked away for future meals. Many of these veggies were grown in our backyard. As the eldest child, I was in charge of the garden, and some of the first vegetables I planted were carrots. After tilling the soil and making rows, I'd drop a few of the tiny seeds, at 3- or 4-inch intervals, cover them with dirt, and wait. A few weeks later, I would thin the crop by pulling up the infant roots, rubbing the dirt off, and then quickly eating them.

One year, I ate so many of these little seedlings that my hands turned orange from the beta-carotene (a nutrient that gives carrots their color)! A friend's mother noticed my hands and asked if I'd been eating carrots.

Back in the precomputer days of my childhood, I got my nutrition information from the families who lived on my street. For instance: My friends and I knew that carrots were supposed to be good for your eyes. Because all of us wanted super vision, guess what we munched on? The mother of one of my friends regularly used mashed potatoes to stop diarrhea and soothe the digestive tract. Another applied slices of red beet for about an hour to help get rid of pimples, boils, and ingrown hair. Beets are known as a purifying vegetable, and after the beet slices were removed skin conditions would always seem much better. Another neighbor would make astringent parsnip-barley water tea to cure urinary tract infections—and there were so many other cases where roots were used to soothe and heal a variety of conditions.

When I got to high school, I first experienced jicama—sparkled with lime juice and dusted with chili powder—at a classmate's *abuelita*'s home, while the Northern European favorite celeriac (enjoyed in my father's family pureed with butter) was part of a "foreign food" day at school!

I was beginning to see that these humble, misshapen, and often homely ingredients—which literally grew underground—were

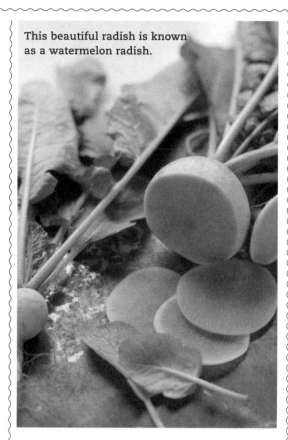

This beautiful radish is known as a watermelon radish.

used by people all over the world as food, as medicine, and even as a source of cultural identity.

A perfect example of food and cultural identity comes from my husband Richard's Sicilian family, who gave me my first taste of rutabaga, which they affectionately, if mistakenly, call a turnip. Every Thanksgiving and Christmas they purchase the largest rutabaga they can find. They peel and boil it, and serve it with ziti for the holiday. The rutabaga, also known as a swede, is not native to Sicily (its origin can be traced to northern Europe), but it is beloved by Richard's family, nonetheless. Why? Because they associate it both with their arrival in America and as an integral, very American part of that most American of feasts, Thanksgiving dinner.

The first year that Richard and I cooked our own holiday meal, he watched me carefully unpack the provisions I'd just purchased from the store. "Where is the turnip?" he asked. After correcting him ("Don't you mean *rutabaga?*"), I trudged back to the produce shelves and picked up the largest one I could find. Twenty-three years later, the rutabaga is an established part of our holiday meals and something I know our three sons will pass on to their families.

Family and tradition—roots have connotations of both. Roots can also be glamorous and esoteric, as I discovered when I was a young adult and had just entered the food world at the Natural Gourmet Culinary Institute. As I was assisting the chef instructor, who was teaching a class on macrobiotic food, she emptied a bag of burdock, salsify, and sunchoke roots and asked me to clean them. I had never seen any of them before! I always think of macrobiotics as the "Paleo" of the 1970s and 1980s—a style of eating based on the Taoist principle of the balance of yin and yang and advocating the consumption of alkalizing foods as well as root vegetables, greens, and brown rice with small amounts of fish and soy.

As I soon learned, burdock, which looks like a brown, leathery carrot, has a dense, satisfying texture and is used in Traditional Chinese Medicine to heal skin conditions, stimulate hair growth, and purify the blood.

Salsify, also known as the "oyster plant" because of its flavor, is related to the dandelion. It is long and skinny, with a brown skin that you peel to reveal the creamy ivory flesh beneath.

Sunchokes—sometimes called Jerusalem artichokes—aren't related to artichokes at all, but, like artichokes, are members of the sunflower family. These knobby little roots have a nutty texture and taste slightly of celery. They are delicious when roasted, but also taste good when they are pureed or added to soups and stews.

If these roots are new to you, you'll learn more about them—and many other roots, too—in the pages ahead. As I wrote this book, I learned a few wonderful things about these superfoods firsthand:

- The difference between a good bowl of chicken soup and a great one is the addition of parsnips. The earthy, almost herbal taste of this root adds another level of flavor to the usual recipe for chicken soup, and gives it depth and a bright-tasting finish.

- Jicama slices are a fantastic replacement for tortilla chips and crackers. Simply cut one of these roots into slices and use them as a dipper for guacamole, hummus, salsa, or even nut butter. Jicama also boasts a generous amount of iron, to help your blood stores and boost energy levels.

- Cooking a pale-colored root, such as rutabaga, then pureeing and stirring it into a bowl of mashed potatoes is the easiest way to "fancy up" the humble spud (as well as give it a boost of additional nutrition). Use whatever ratios you like, but my favorite is 50 percent potato and 50 percent rutabaga. A nice extra is a dusting of cayenne powder or sweet paprika, or a sprinkle of herbs as a garnish.

- When I was in my twenties, I was told that eating burdock—which is known in Traditional Chinese Medicine as a beautifying food—a couple of times a week during the autumn and winter would keep my skin clear and wrinkle-free and my hair thick and lustrous. I'm now in my late forties, and both my skin and hair are in great shape.

- When I am feeling run-down and fatigued, I add beets to my morning juice and daily

salad. In Traditional Chinese Medicine and Ayurveda, beets are considered a blood-building vegetable, and I always feel stronger after I have eaten them.

Not a day goes by that I don't enjoy at least one root. I throw a bit of beet, carrot, or celeriac into my juicer for my morning drink, which leaves me feeling refreshed and clear-headed. I often munch on a few baby carrots (usually with hummus or almond butter) mid-morning. For lunch, I enjoy a salad with grated turnip and radish, or a soup with lentils, parsnips, and sweet potatoes. My afternoon snack is often a few slices of jicama dipped into my favorite avocado-coconut dip (for the recipe, check out *Coconut: The Complete Guide to the World's Most Versatile Superfood)*. One of my favorite dinnertime side dishes is roasted burdock, salsify, sunchoke, potato, and rutabaga. Some days, I toss roots in coconut oil, with a dusting of allspice and thyme, for a Jamaican-themed side. Other times, I might try extra virgin olive oil, oregano, and basil, for a more Italian-style dish.

I've even been known to sauté a few cups of mixed roots or a leftover baked sweet potato with a few cloves of garlic, and then puree it all with a cup or two of chicken or veggie stock, to make a delicious soup. Even while writing this, I'm pureeing my latest impromptu batch of root veggie bisque.

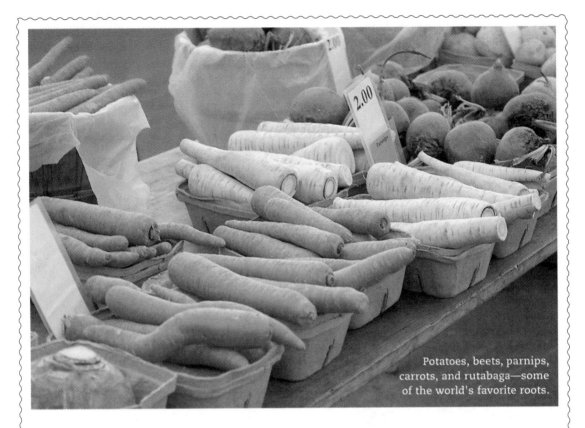

Potatoes, beets, parnips, carrots, and rutabaga—some of the world's favorite roots.

Indeed, roots are the easiest, most agreeable vegetables on earth to prepare, and they are powerful forces for good: They are nourishing and sustaining; they help prevent and heal disease; and they are compatible with almost any method of cooking, from simple boiling to baking and roasting. As ingredients, roots take a leading role in stews, soups, and casseroles; they supply garnishes for salads; and they add sweetness or crunch to other foods. Also, roots always play nicely, whether you cook them in oil or fat, douse them with sauce or dressing, toss them with herbs, or dust them with spices.

If you take away only one thing from this book, let it be this: Roots are healthy, delicious, and versatile superfoods that you can use in myriad ways to bring great flavors and textures to meals and snacks every day!

Here's to your health!

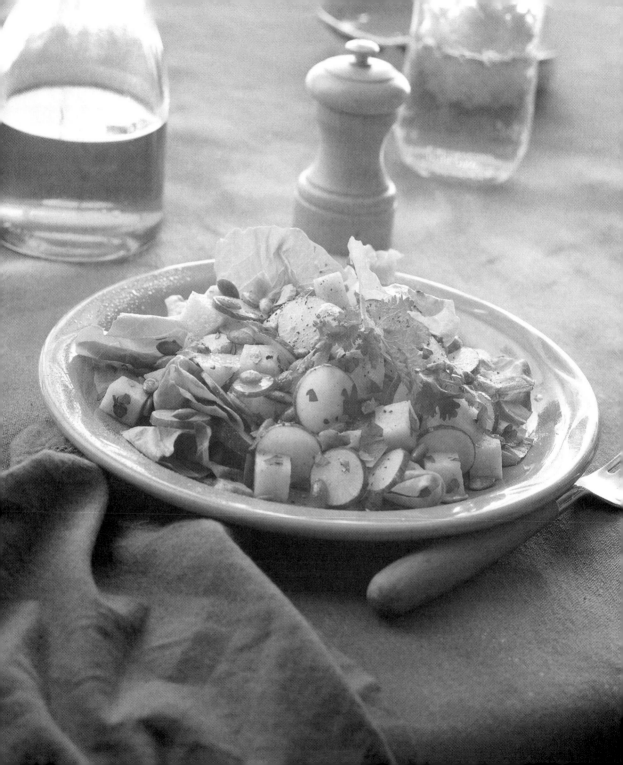

CHAPTER 1

ALL ABOUT THE ROOTS

Humans have eaten roots since the beginning of time. Hearty, filling, nourishing, and relatively easy to find—even during times of famine and other extreme conditions—root vegetables have long been humankind's dietary backbone.

One reason for this is their intrepid nature: Roots grow on every continent but Antarctica. Sandy soil, loamy soil, clay-like soil. Moist conditions, dry conditions, perfect conditions, imperfect conditions. Winter, spring, summer, fall. Wherever you are, there is a root that will grow for you.

Once pulled from the ground, root vegetables last without much work. Pack them in cool sand or earth and tuck them away in a dark cellar and there they will stay, happily, for months at a time. Consider that refrigeration—as we know it today—didn't arrive on the culinary scene until the 1920s, and you can see the importance of vegetables that last and last.

And while hardiness is important, so is nutrition. Roots boast generous amounts of fiber, phytonutrients, vitamins, minerals, and other nutrients. This is no unimportant feat when you consider that roots can be stored and enjoyed throughout the cold season when other plant food may be unavailable.

Roots are also yummy! Whether you like your veggies sweet or crunchy, mild or with a bitter kick, there are a number of roots to suit your taste buds. Furthermore, roots are versatile. Slice raw radishes into a salad or roast them as a side dish. Shred carrots into a salad or puree and add them to a smoothie. Juice the greens of carrots, turnips, radishes, and beets or toss them in a pot with garlic and a bit of oil for an easy, economical side dish. You can bake, braise, slice, dice, eat them whole, juice, or shred them raw—there are dozens of ways to enjoy each root vegetable.

In these days of rising food costs, roots offer one of the most affordable and nutrient-dense foods on the planet. Unlike $18-a-pound chia seeds and cartons of $10 organic blueberries, a pound of carrots, radishes, or parsnips—organic or not—is generally available for under a buck. Five-pound bags of potatoes or cassava are routinely only a few dollars. And giant

OPPOSITE: **Jicama, Radish, and Pepita Salad (page 90)**

globes of celeriac, rutabaga, and jicama hover around a dollar. Even the more exotic roots—burdock, salsify, sunchokes—are only a few dollars a pound, much cheaper than their green leafy brethren.

Are you ready to learn more about making this important superfood family part of your daily diet? Start here, by getting to know the roots we feature in *Roots: The Complete Guide to the Underground Superfood.*

BEETS

NUTRITIONAL PROFILE PER SERVING (1 CUP RAW; 136 G)

Calories: 58
Fiber: 3.8 g
Protein: 2.2 g
Vitamin C: 6.7 mg
Beta-carotene: 28 mcg
Betaine: 175 mg
Choline: 8.2 mg
Folate: 148 mcg
Manganese: 0.4 mg
Omega-3 fatty acids: 6.8 mg
Phytosterols: 34.0 mg
Potassium: 442 mg

ROLE IN SUPPORTING HEALTH

IMPROVES PHYSICAL STAMINA: Consuming beets or beet juice the day of a big race or game is common among many athletes who believe that the high levels of dietary nitrate in beets can help lower blood pressure, oxygenate the muscles, and prevent physical fatigue. A recent study from the University of Exeter's Sport and Health Sciences Department found that 2–3 hours after ingesting 70 milliliters of beet juice, test subjects enjoyed the greatest benefits. These benefits, which included a feeling of energy as well as lowered blood pressure, gradually disappeared over the course of 12 hours.

INCREASES ATHLETIC PERFORMANCE: In another study, performed at the University of West Scotland, competitive cyclists who enjoyed 70 milliliters of beet juice before cycling improved performance by 2.8 percent (11 seconds) in a 4-kilometer bicycle time trial and by 2.7 percent (45 seconds) in 16.1-kilometer time trial.

SLOWS THE PROGRESSION OF DEMENTIA: Researchers at Wake Forest University have found that drinking juice from beets can improve oxygenation to the brain, slowing the progression of dementia in older adults who have begun to show signs of the disease. Blood flow to certain areas of the brain decreases with age, which can lead to lowered cognitive function and possible dementia. The nitrates in beets can improve the blood flow and oxygenation to these areas that are lacking.

SUPPORTS HEART HEALTH AND HEALTHY BLOOD PRESSURE: In a study of 30 healthy men and women performed by researchers at the Baker IDI Heart and Diabetes Institute in Melbourne, Australia, beets were found to reduce systolic blood pressure by an average of five points within 2 hours of consumption. Other studies have also found beets to be heart-friendly: A 2008 study by a team of British researchers published in *Hypertension* examined the effects of ingesting 500 milliliters of beet juice in healthy volunteers and found that blood pressure was significantly lowered after ingestion.

GENERAL INFORMATION

PURCHASING: Purchase beets that are firm and heavy for their size with no cuts or weepy spots. I like to buy beets with the greens because it gives me an indication of how fresh the beets are *and* I get to enjoy the greens—just cook as you would chard.

STORAGE: Store beets unwashed in your vegetable crisper, either loose or in a paper bag or special produce bag. If your beets come with greens, remove those and store them separately.

USAGE: Use within a week. Beets can be enjoyed raw, juiced, or cooked in any way that you'd like.

BOTANICAL BACKGROUND: Beets are the taproot of the *Beta vulgaris* plant, which is a member of the Amaranthaceae family.

HISTORY: Beets are thought to originate in the Mediterranean as a domesticated offspring of the wild sea beet that grows along the coast of the Mediterranean Sea. Beets have been found by archeologists at Neolithic sites throughout Europe, as well in the burial chambers of pyramids at Thebes, Egypt.

GROWING INFORMATION: This biennial plant grows best in sunny, well-drained areas.

THINGS TO BE AWARE OF: Even one serving of beets or beet juice can give your urine a pink tinge.

STEPHANIE'S FAVORITE USES: I love beets in so many ways that it is hard to choose a favorite beet dish, but if you twist my arm I'd have to say that I enjoy beets shredded raw and dressed with lime juice, cumin, and cilantro as a fast side salad.

THE NUTRIENTS IN ROOTS: HOW MUCH DO YOU NEED?

Name a nutrient—any nutrient—and chances are good that different people, of different ages, life stages, and genders, need different amounts of it. This is why the United States Department of Agriculture has created nutritional guidelines for most nutrients in the form of RDA (recommended dietary allowance) or AI (adequate intake). Here is a list of nutrients that root vegetables are known for, along with the USDA's intake suggestions, where they exist. Some nutrients do not yet have an RDA; in these cases, the lowest generally suggested dose is given. *Note*: The USDA breaks down recommended dietary allowances into very narrow groups, as well as offering suggestions for larger, more general groups. Here, I share with you the amounts recommended for those nutrients.

FIBER
Helps move food through the stomach and intestines and adds bulk to stool. Fiber has been found to lower the risk of colorectal cancer and other gastrointestinal cancers.

> men, over the age of 18: **38 g**
> women, over the age of 18: **25 g**
> pregnant women: **28 g**

PROTEIN
An important building block of bones, muscles, cartilage, skin, and blood. Responsible for helping the body build and repair itself.

> men, over the age of 18: **56 g**
> women, over the age of 18: **26 g**
> pregnant women: **71 g**

VITAMIN A
Plays an important role in the normal formation and maintenance of the heart, lungs, kidneys, and other vital organs. Vitamin A is needed for new cell growth and healthy skin, hair, and tissues.

> men, over the age of 18: **900 IUs**
> women, over the age of 18: **700 IUs**
> pregnant women: **770 IUs**

VITAMIN B6
The body uses vitamin B6 for more than a hundred enzyme reactions involved in metabolism, as well as brain development and immune function in utero and during infancy. Also called pyridoxine, it converts food into glucose, which is used to produce energy and make neurotransmitters. These neurotransmitters carry signals from one nerve cell to another.

> men, over the age of 18: **1.3 mg**
> women, over the age of 18: **1.3 mg**
> pregnant women: **1.9 mg**

VITAMIN C
Makes collagen, an important protein in skin, cartilage, tendons, ligaments, and blood vessels, as well as helping heal wounds and form scar tissue. Vitamin C also supports functioning of the immune system.

> men, over the age of 18: **90 mg**
> women, over the age of 18: **75 mg**
> pregnant women: **85 mg**

VITAMIN E

An important antioxidant vitamin that improves immune system function, helps lower the risk of cancer, and reduces blood cholesterol levels.

> men, over the age of 18: **15 mg**
> women, over the age of 18: **15 mg**
> pregnant women: **15 mg**

VITAMIN K

Known best for its role in healthy blood clotting, this vitamin also helps halt age-related bone loss and can prevent and minimize the severity of dementia, tooth decay, and infectious diseases such as pneumonia.

> men, over the age of 18: **120 g**
> women, over the age of 18: **90 g**
> pregnant women: **90 g**

ALPHA-CAROTENE

A member of the carotene family, alpha-carotene is present in many types of berries. It is a powerful antioxidant that helps prevent the breakdown of body tissue due to free-radical damage.

> men, over the age of 18: **24 mcg**
> women, over the age of 18: **24 mcg**
> pregnant women: **24 mcg**

BETA-CAROTENE

A member of the carotene family, beta-carotene plays a significant role in preventing heart disease, viral infections, cataracts, and cancer and reducing the severity if they do develop.

> men, over the age of 18: **3,000 IU**
> women, over the age of 18: **2,310 IU**
> pregnant women: **2,310 IU**

CALCIUM

In addition to its well-known role as a bone and tooth builder, calcium helps muscles move and nerves carry messages between the brain and other parts of the body.

> men, over the age of 18: **1,000 mg**
> women, over the age of 18: **1,000 mg**
> pregnant women: **1,000 mg**

CHOLINE

This micronutrient helps the body with nerve signaling, maintains cell membranes, and transports triglycerides from the liver.

> men, over the age of 18: **250 mg**
> women, over the age of 18: **250 mg**
> pregnant women: **250 mg**

FLUORIDE

Helps keep teeth and bones strong and dense.

> men, over the age of 18: **0.05 mg**
> women, over the age of 18: **0.05 mg**
> pregnant women: **0.05 mg**

FOLATE

Needed for the formation of red and white blood cells in bone marrow, the conversion of carbohydrates into energy, and the production of DNA and RNA.

> men, over the age of 18: **400 g**
> women, over the age of 18: **400 g**
> pregnant women: **600 g**

IRON
Helps the body create red blood cells, store and transport oxygen to tissues, and protect cells against the damaging effects of free radicals.

> men, over the age of 18: **8 mg**
> women, over the age of 18: **18 mg**
> pregnant women: **27 mg**

LUTEIN
Helps maintain vision and helps prevent diseases of the eye.

> men, over the age of 18: **10 mg**
> women, over the age of 18: **10 mg**
> pregnant women: **6 mg**

LYCOPENE
This antioxidant may help reduce the risk of developing cardiovascular disease by reducing LDL ("bad") cholesterol and lowering blood pressure. It also helps prevent cancer.

> men, over the age of 18: **15 mg**
> women, over the age of 18: **15 mg**
> pregnant women: **15 mg**

MAGNESIUM
A mineral responsible for many biochemical functions in the body, including regulating the heart rhythm and supporting the function of nerve cells. Magnesium is a major electrolyte that helps maintain proper fluid levels in the body and helps regulate muscle function.

> men, over the age of 18: **400 mg**
> women, over the age of 18: **310 mg**
> pregnant women: **350 mg**

MANGANESE
This mineral is involved in processing cholesterol, carbohydrates, and protein. It helps the body form skin and bone cells and helps regulate blood sugar.

> men, over the age of 18: **2.3 mg**
> women, over the age of 18: **1.8mg**
> pregnant women: **2 mg**

NIACIN
Also known as vitamin B3, niacin performs many roles in the body. It helps break down carbohydrates, fats, and proteins and convert them into energy. It also plays a role in producing hormones in the adrenal glands and removing harmful chemicals from the liver.

> men, over the age of 18: **16 mg**
> women, over the age of 18: **14 mg**
> pregnant women: **18 mg**

OMEGA-3 FATTY ACIDS
Help lower the risk of heart disease, support joint health, and improve the skin. Additionally, they support brain health by reducing the risk of depression and dementia.

> men, over the age of 18: **250 mg**
> women, over the age of 18: **250 mg**
> pregnant women: **250 mg**

PHOSPHORUS
After calcium, phosphorous is the second most abundant mineral in the body. It helps create strong bones and teeth.

> men, over the age of 18: **700 mg**
> women, over the age of 18: **700 mg**
> pregnant women: **700 mg**

PHYTOSTEROLS
Help lower blood cholesterol levels and strengthen the immune system.

> men, over the age of 18: **1.3 g**
> women, over the age of 18: **1.3 g**
> pregnant women: **0.2 g**

POTASSIUM
Controls blood pressure and reduces the risk of heart disease by helping the body conduct electricity, which is crucial to heart function and muscle contraction.

> men, over the age of 18: **4.7 g**
> women, over the age of 18: **4.7 g**
> pregnant women: **4.7 g**

RIBOFLAVIN
Also called vitamin B2, riboflavin defends the body against free radicals, which damage cells and contribute to aging.

> men, over the age of 18: **1.3 mg**
> women, over the age of 18: **1.1 mg**
> pregnant women: **1.4 mg**

SELENIUM
Helps thyroid function and strengthens the immune system.

> men, over the age of 18: **55 mcg**
> women, over the age of 18: **55 mcg**
> pregnant women: **60 mcg**

THIAMINE
Known as vitamin B1, thiamine helps the nervous system function properly, strengthens the immune system, and is needed for brain function.

> men, over the age of 18: **1.2 mg**
> women, over the age of 18: **1.1 mg**
> pregnant women: **1.4 mg**

ZINC
Builds a strong immune system and is used by the body in wound healing, blood clotting, and thyroid function.

> men, over the age of 18: **11 mg**
> women, over the age of 18: **8 mg**
> pregnant women: **11 mg**

BURDOCK

NUTRITIONAL PROFILE PER SERVING (1 CUP RAW; 120 G)

Calories: 85
Fiber: 3.9 g
Protein: 1.8 g
Vitamin B6: 0.3 mcg
Vitamin C: 3.5 mg
Betaine: 0.2 mg
Choline: 14 mg
Folate: 27.1 mcg
Magnesium: 44.8 mg
Manganese: 0.3 mcg
Omega-3 fatty acids: 2.4 mg
Potassium: 363 mg

ROLE IN SUPPORTING HEALTH

REDUCES INFLAMMATION IN ARTHRITIS PATIENTS: Burdock has long been a folk remedy for inflammatory conditions such as arthritis, gout, and hypertension. Studies support this. One of these, performed in 2014 by researchers from Tabriz University in Iran, found that burdock significantly reduced the inflammation in individuals with osteoarthritis of the knees. Thirty-six test subjects—men and women, all with arthritis, all within the 50–70 age range—were split into two equal groups. For 42 days, one group received burdock tea three times a day. The other received a placebo. At the end of the study, the burdock group showed markedly lower oxidative stress and inflammation than the placebo group.

ENHANCES LIBIDO: In traditional Chinese medicine, burdock is celebrated for its ability to enhance one's sex drive. Researchers at Shandong University in China put this old wives' tale to the test by giving it to male rats. One group of rats received a placebo, one received Viagra, and one received burdock extract. While the Viagra group showed the most aggressive sexual behavior (mounting, intromission, and ejaculation frequency were recorded, as well as the number of female rats that became pregnant by these male test rats) and the highest measured testosterone levels, the burdock group was a close second. Researchers believe that high levels of flavonoids, saponins, lignans, and alkaloids in burdock may be what enhanced the sexual activity of the rats.

HELPS WITH WEIGHT LOSS AND WEIGHT MAINTENANCE: In a study done by researchers at Kyung Hee University in Seoul, South Korea, obese mice on a high-fat diet were given supplements of arctiin, a lingan found in burdock, or a placebo. After 8 days, the mice given arctiin showed lower levels of cholesterol in their blood and experienced 26 percent lower body weight than the placebo group.

REDUCES BREAST CANCER RISK:
Researchers at the University of Agriculture in Faisalabad, Pakistan, recently reviewed over 200 studies of plant foods that lower the risk of cancer and have antitumor properties. After looking at the data, researchers determined that several foods could help prevent cancer, including burdock root, which they suggested people eat weekly. Results were published in the May 2016 issue of *Saudi Pharmacology Journal*. Burdock has been utilized as a helpful traditional remedy historically for treatment of breast tumors, malignant melanoma, lymphoma, and ovarian, pancreatic, and bladder cancers. It is said to reduce cancer pain, lessen tumor size, and enhance the survival phase. Among the suggested explanations is that burdock root consists of polyphenol antioxidants and flavonoids, and they may suppress tumor development. Normal body cells are protected from toxic substances, and cell mutation is prevented by extracts of the root. Burdock contains the important active ingredient known as tannin, a phenolic compound. It stimulates macrophage action, limits cancer propagation, and retains immune-modulatory properties.

GENERAL INFORMATION

PURCHASING: Burdock root is covered with a very thin, slightly fuzzy brown skin that makes it appear to be covered by a layer of dirt. Look for firm, unbroken roots without weepy spots. Avoid roots that look withered or bendy. Roots that are about 1 inch in diameter and no more than 18 inches in length will be the most tender. You can also purchase dried burdock, either sliced or chopped. This can be reconstituted in liquid.

STORAGE: Burdock root can be stored for up to 2 months in a cool, dry, dark place. I like to place it dry (do not wash before storage, as the root will develop mold) in a root cellar or wrapped in a towel, placed in an airtight container, and stored, refrigerated, in the back of the vegetable crisper. If the root feels limp, you can plunge it into ice water for a minute or two to firm it up.

USAGE: Right before using, brush burdock vigorously with a wet vegetable brush to remove the brown skin. Burdock can be eaten raw, sliced or diced into soups and stews, braised, roasted, boiled and mashed, fried, and even shredded raw into salads. Because burdock oxidizes very quickly, have a bowl of acidulated water (water with a few drops of lemon juice or vinegar or wine) available and drop pieces of the root into it as you peel and cut them. This will keep them light colored until you are ready to cook them.

BOTANICAL BACKGROUND: Burdock is a taproot that is a member of the Asteracae family, which includes other root vegetables such as sunchokes and yacon.

HISTORY: Known as gobo or beggar's root in Japan, burdock has been an important medicinal and culinary vegetable in Asia since the tenth century. The leaves and roots are used to heal skin conditions, and the root is prized as a diuretic, blood purifier, anti-inflammatory (which helps relieve the pain of arthritis and joint conditions), and cancer preventative.

GROWING INFORMATION: Burdock grows wild in temperate areas of Asia, Europe, and North America alongside roads, in backyards, and in vacant lots. It enjoys mild weather, some sun, and slightly sandy soil, but will grow in cooler weather, partial shade, and heavier soils, too. It is traditionally harvested in September.

THINGS TO BE AWARE OF: Burdock's pretty purple flowers grow into burrs that are so tenacious, birds can become ensnared in them. These burrs were the inspiration—indeed, the actual model—for Velcro.

STEPHANIE'S FAVORITE USES: I love burdock cubed, tossed with sesame oil, and roasted—as much as I love it sliced thin and fried into chips.

CARROTS

NUTRITIONAL PROFILE PER SERVING (1 CUP RAW; 128 G)

> *Calories: 52*
> *Fiber: 3.6 g*
> *Protein: 1.2 g*
> *Vitamin A: 21,383 IU*
> *Vitamin B6: 24.3 mg*
> *Vitamin C: 7.6 mg*
> *Vitamin K: 16.9 mcg*
> *Alpha-carotene: 44,451 mcg*
> *Beta-carotene: 10,605 mcg*
> *Betaine: 0.5 mg*
> *Choline: 12 mg*
> *Lutein: 328 mcg*
> *Lycopene: 1.3 mcg*
> *Manganese: 0.2 mg*
> *Omega-3 fatty acids: 3 mg*
> *Potassium: 410 mg*

ROLE IN SUPPORTING HEALTH

REDUCE THE RISK OF PROSTATE CANCER: A team of researchers from Zhejiang University in China examined a number of past studies on the effect of carrot consumption on prostate cancer. They found that for each 10-gram serving of carrots that a man consumed, there was an almost 1 percent reduction in his chance of developing prostate cancer. It is believed that the carotenes and phytonutrients in carrots are what help ward off cancer.

IMPROVES HEART HEALTH: Researchers from Texas A&M University gave 18 test subjects a 16-ounce serving of fresh-squeezed carrot juice every day for 3 months. Weight, fasting blood sugar levels, blood pressure, and blood cholesterol levels were taken at the begin and the end of the study. The findings? While consuming carrot juice daily did not lead to any change in weight or blood sugar levels, it did increase the levels of antioxidants in the blood and helped suppress free radical levels in the blood, both of which in turn help keep the cardiovascular system strong and healthy.

HELPS PREVENT CARDIOVASCULAR DISEASE: A 10-year study from Wageningen University in the Netherlands found that carrots reduced the risk of cardiovascular disease. Researchers followed 20,069 men and women, aged 20–65 years, for a decade, encouraging them to eat fruits and vegetables with their meals. During 10 years of follow-up, 245 incident cases of cardiovascular disease were documented. For each 25 grams of carrots an individual ate each day, the greater the decrease in cardiovascular disease. Those who ate the most carrots—50–75 grams or more daily—cut their risk of heart disease by 32 percent.

PREVENTS GLAUCOMA: Researchers at the University of California at Los Angeles studied 1,155 women over age 65. The risk of glaucoma was lowered by 64 percent in women who ate more than two servings a week of carrots compared with those who ate less than one serving a week. Glaucoma is damage to the optic nerve often associated with excessive pressure inside the eye.

GENERAL INFORMATION

PURCHASING: Look for firm, nicely colored roots with no weepy spots, bruises, or wrinkling. I like purchasing carrots with their green tops (make sure they are bright and fresh-looking), which I then remove and run through the juicer for my morning green drinks.

STORAGE: Place carrots, unwashed, in a paper or plastic storage bag in the vegetable crisper drawer of your refrigerator. They will keep up to a month.

USAGE: Carrots can be pickled, juiced, eaten raw, grated raw into salad, cut into sticks, sliced into salads and other dishes—even boiled, baked, braised, or sautéed.

BOTANICAL BACKGROUND: Carrots are part of the Apicae (also called the Umbelliferae) family, along with botanical cousins celery and parsley.

HISTORY: Garden carrots as we know them today are believed to have originated in the tenth century from wild carrots that grew in what is now Afghanistan. The name *carota* for the garden carrot was first used in the Roman writings of Athenaeus in 200 CE.

GROWING INFORMATION: Carrot seeds are incredibly tiny and must be sown in finely tilled, lump-free, well-drained soil. A cool-weather crop, carrots like full sun and will tolerate partial shade. They do like moderate weather—nothing too hot or too cold. The traditional harvest time for carrots is in September or early fall.

THINGS TO BE AWARE OF: Baby carrots—those lunch box, snack-time darlings—are not actually immature carrots at all. They are pieces that have broken off large carrots and have been polished into the famous fingerling shape we all know and love.

STEPHANIE'S FAVORITE USES: Carrots are one of the workhorses of my kitchen. I do so many things with them, but my absolutely favorite use for them is juicing them with a large amount of lemon.

CASSAVA

NUTRITIONAL PROFILE PER SERVING (1 CUP COOKED; 206 G)

Calories: 330
Fiber: 3.7 g
Protein: 2.8 g
Vitamin C: 42 mg
Beta-carotene: 16.5 mcg
Betaine: 0.8 mg
Choline: 48.8 mg
Folate: 56 mcg
Niacin: 1.8 mg
Omega-3 fatty acids: 35 mg
Thiamin: 0.3 mcg

ROLE IN SUPPORTING HEALTH

REDUCES THE RISK OF STROKE: A serving of cassava provides around 70 percent of your daily requirement for vitamin C, an antioxidant with strong anti-inflammatory properties. Researchers at Tokyo Medical and Dental University followed 880 men and 1,241 women aged 40 years and older who had never suffered a stroke. They were first examined in 1977 with a final follow-up examination in 1997. The findings? Individuals who had the highest blood serum levels of vitamin C had a 29 percent lower risk of stroke than those with the lowest serum levels of vitamin C. Additionally, the risk of stroke in those who consumed vitamin C–rich vegetables 6–7 days of the week was 54 percent lower than in those who consumed vitamin C–rich vegetables 0–2 days of the week. Similar studies have been performed elsewhere, including a 10-year research project by the University of Cambridge in the United Kingdom among 20,649 originally stroke-free men and women aged 40–79. Similarly, the 25 percent of study subjects with the highest plasma vitamin C levels had a 42 percent lower risk of stroke over the decade compared to the 25 percent who had the lowest vitamin C levels.

HELPS PREVENT CANCER AND SHRINK TUMOR CELLS: Researchers from the University of Liège in Belgium found that extract of cassava contained high polyphenol and flavonoid content, groups of nutrients known to help prevent cancer and shrink tumors. Researchers looked at cassava extract's ability to shrink cancer cells in vitro. Two servings of cooked cassava per week could offer the same protection.

PROVIDES CANCER-FIGHTING SAPONINS: Cassava is a rich source of saponins, a substance that protects plants from birds and insects by creating a bitter-tasting, soapy coating. Scientists at Tianjin University in China found that these saponins also possess significant cancer-preventative abilities when tested in vitro on cancer cells.

CASSAVA ROOT FOR TWINS? When I was trying to conceive my second child, my West Indian friends encouraged my husband and me to eat cassava, saying it would make us more fertile. Some even suggested it would help us conceive twins. In researching this, I found that many natural fertility supplements are either based on, or contain, cassava. While I still am looking for a scientific study on this, I continue to hear cassava suggested to people trying to conceive.

GENERAL INFORMATION

PURCHASING: You can find cassava root in the produce department of well-stocked supermarkets and markets that carry West Indian and South American foods. If you're having trouble finding it, look for it under the name manioc or yuca, names it also goes by. (You may even find it mistakenly called yucca, after the hardy plant that grows in the deserts of the U.S.). Roots should be firm and heavy with a slightly shiny brown, bark-like skin. The root is often coated in a protective wax by growers.

STORAGE: Cassava is not anywhere near as hearty as other roots; refrigerate it unwashed in your veggie crisper and use it within three days. If you cannot use it right away, peel it, cut it in chunks, boil until just firm, drain, cool, and put parboiled chunks in a freezer-safe container. Freeze for up to three months.

USAGE: Cassava must be cooked before being eaten, as the raw root contains a cyanide-like plant chemical that dissipates with heat and is neutralized. Peel the root and cut or chop into chunks before boiling or baking. Cassava has a slightly gelatinous finish which some people love (and others loathe).

BOTANICAL BACKGROUND: Cassava is a member of the Euphorbiaceae family and grows in a number of tropical countries, including those in the West Indies, Southeast Asia, Central and South America, and Africa.

HISTORY: In 2008, 230 million tons of cassava were grown. In many countries, such as Ghana, it makes up 30 percent or more of the local diet. But cassava is not a fad food—it has a long culinary history. Cassava has been found in Central American ruins, including the 1,400-year-old Mayan site Joya de Ceren, in El Salvador. Paintings and pottery depicting the root are also common in the pre-Columbian indigenous art of Central and South America.

GROWING INFORMATION: Cassava is the root of a tall tree-like plant that enjoys warmth and sunny climates, but beyond that, it is an adaptable plant, tolerating poor soils that can be acidic or alkaline. It is well-known for its ability to thrive in droughts, which makes it a favorite of African farmers. While it does grow wild in rainforests and in other temperate areas, it is most often seen growing on plantations.

THINGS TO BE AWARE OF: Raw cassava contains two "antinutrients," linamarin and lotaustralin, which are a type of natural cyanide. While these can cause goiter, ataxia, or coma when consumed raw, they are neutralized when the cassava is boiled, baked, or cooked. Cassava is the third-largest source of food carbohydrates in the tropics, after rice and corn, a diet staple for more than half a billion people. It is definitely worth eating. You just need to cook it first.

STEPHANIE'S FAVORITE USES: Tapioca pudding, of course! Made with coconut milk and garnished with berries and chopped nuts.

CASSAVA: DID YOU KNOW?

- Africa accounts for more than 50 percent of world cassava production.

- Cassava is grown commercially in Indonesia, Malaysia, the Philippines, and parts of Africa.

- Cassava originated in the Amazon Basin region of Brazil. In the sixteenth century Portuguese sailors brought it to Africa.

CELERIAC

NUTRITIONAL PROFILE PER SERVING
(1 CUP RAW; 156 G)

Calories: 65
Fiber: 2.8 g
Protein: 2.3 g
Vitamin B6: 0.3 mg
Vitamin C: 13 mg
Vitamin K: 64 mcg
Calcium: 67 mg
Choline: 12 mg
Lutein: 1.6 mcg
Manganese: 0.2 mg
Phosphorus: 179 mg
Potassium: 468 mg

ROLE IN SUPPORTING HEALTH

INHIBITS BREAST CANCER CELL GROWTH: In several studies on animals and in vitro, researchers have found that apigenin, a phytonutrient found in celeriac, inhibits breast cancer cell growth. One of these studies, performed by researchers from the Indiana University School of Medicine, looked at cancerous cells that were resistant to anticancer drugs tamoxifen and fulvestrant. It was found that in low concentrations, apigenin stimulated healthy cell growth. In high doses, apigenin both stimulated healthy cell growth and inhibited the growth of cancerous cells.

STOPS COGNITIVE DECLINE: In another study on apigenin, this one performed by researchers at Central South University in China, it was found that apigenin improved learning and cognitive function and reversed cognitive decline in rats that had diabetes-associated cognitive decline. Researchers believe it works by increasing brain chemicals that improve cognitive ability.

HELPS KEEP BONES STRONG AND PREVENTS OSTEOPOROSIS: A serving of celeriac provides about 34 percent of an adult's daily requirement of vitamin K, a nutrient that helps create and maintain bone mass. One study, from Tufts University in Boston, measured the spine and hip bone density of 112 men and 1,479 women, aged 29 through 86. While men with low and high vitamin K levels showed little difference in bone density, women were more affected by vitamin K levels: Those who consumed less than 70.2 mcg per day had significantly lower bone mass density than those who had 309 mcg per day.

GENERAL INFORMATION

PURCHASING: Also labeled in markets as celery root, celeriac may look hairy (these "hairs" are actually small roots) and a bit dirty. Pay no mind to that; what you want to look for is a firm, heavy-feeling root that has no weepy spots or cracks and is free of withering or wrinkling. If the leaves are attached, they should look fresh and green.

STORAGE: Store unwashed in a storage bag in the vegetable drawer of your refrigerator, where it can stay for over a month. If the root is sold with its greens, remove those and store them (also unwashed) in a separate bag in the vegetable drawer.

USAGE: To use celeriac, peel away the tough, ridged skin and slice or chop as needed. If not cooking with celeriac immediately, drop pieces into acidulated water (water with a few drops of lemon juice or vinegar) to preserve its color, as slices will brown quickly. The stalks and leaves can be used as you would celery. Celeriac can be juiced, grated raw into salads and slaws, pickled, boiled, baked, roasted, sautéed, braised, steamed, and fried.

BOTANICAL BACKGROUND: Celeriac is a member of the Apiaceae family (along with carrots, parsley, and dill).

HISTORY: Celeriac has a long and illustrious culinary past, being mentioned in Homer's *Odyssey*, circa 800 BCE, as selinion. Indeed, it's been a favorite with the French, who have enjoyed it since at least the seventeenth century as *céleri-rave rémoulade*, grated and dressed with a mustardy vinaigrette.

GROWING INFORMATION: Celeriac likes cooler temperatures and gentle sun or partial shade. Sow seeds directly into post-frost soil about 6 inches apart. In about 10 weeks, seedlings appear. Soil should be kept barely moist, although the plant does tolerate drier and wetter extremes.

THINGS TO BE AWARE OF: Celeriac is one of a few plants (fennel and celery are two others) that can cause photoreactions of the skin. This occurs when the juice of the plant ends up on the skin and the skin is then exposed to ultraviolet light. The results are dark red splotches on the affected skin; these can take up to a year to disappear and are generally treated with bleaching cream.

STEPHANIE'S FAVORITE USES: I adore celeriac cubed and added to beef stew.

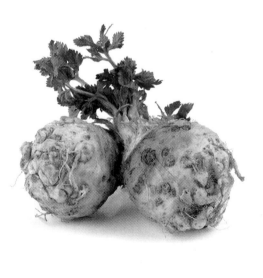

JICAMA

NUTRITIONAL PROFILE PER SERVING
(1 CUP RAW; 120 G)

Calories: 45
Fiber: 6 g
Protein: 0.9 g
Vitamin C: 24 mg
Beta-carotene: 15.6 mcg
Choline: 16.3 mg
Iron: 0.8 mg
Omega-3 fatty acids: 17 mg
Potassium: 180 mg

ROLE IN SUPPORTING HEALTH

LOWERS THE RISK OF COLON CANCER:
Jicama contains large amounts of a type of fiber called inulin, which has been extensively studied for its potential to lower the risk of colorectal cancer. Researchers at Friedrich-Schiller-University in Germany found that inulin fiber, which jicama contains, boasts an antioxidant compound called fructans. In a study on cancerous colon tumors in mice and rats, exposure to these inulin fructans inhibited the growth of tumors and prevented tumors from metastasizing.

HELPS HEAL INTESTINAL DISORDERS SUCH AS IBS AND CROHN'S DISEASE:
In a 2005 study at the University Hospital Vall d'Hebron in Barcelona, Spain, researchers working with rats found that inulin fiber, which jicama contains, improved the metabolic function of the helpful bacteria (aka gut flora) found in the large intestines of rats. It also helped heal the inside of the intestinal wall in the case of ulcerative colitis, inflammatory bowel disease, and Crohn's disease.

LOWERS TRIGLYCERIDE LEVELS:
Researchers at the Université Catholique de Louvain in Brussels tested the ability of inulin to protect overweight rats from high cholesterol levels brought about by overconsumption of simple carbohydrates and fructose. The rats that were lucky to be given 10 percent of their daily calories in inulin-rich foods had 50 percent lower levels of post-meal riglyceride levels than their rodent counterparts who enjoyed the same meal without the inulin.

GENERAL INFORMATION

PURCHASING: Jicamas should be heavy for their size, firm and smooth, with no cuts, blemishes, weepy spots, or withering. In a mainstream U.S. grocery store, you'll find jicamas with other roots or nestled into a section with "South of the border" produce, such as chayote, geneps, and aloe spears.

STORAGE: Place, unwashed, in a cool, dry spot in the pantry or place in the produce drawer of your refrigerator, where it can stay for three weeks or so. The sooner you use

(continued on page 19)

UNUSUAL ROOT VEGETABLES

When I started writing *Roots: The Underground Superfood*, it quickly became clear that there were more edible roots in the world than pages in my book to write about them. Putting on my editor's cap, I sat down to make a few difficult decisions about what to include and what not. My criteria were twofold: The roots that I ultimately included in this book had to be not only nutritious but also relatively easily found in well-stocked markets. Thus, a number of beautiful roots were given a pass. Here are the unusual roots that were allowed to get away.

ARROWROOT: You may have this tropical root (sometimes known as maranta) in your pantry right now in its dried, powdered form; it is a popular culinary thickener. The health world uses arrowroot over wheat flour or cornstarch because arrowroot soothes the stomach and intestines and is easily digestible.

CROSNE: Akin to the sunchoke and native to Japan, the crosne is often referred to as the Japanese artichoke, Chinese artichoke, knot root, or *chorogi*. While it tastes like a sunchoke and can be prepared the same way, crosne looks exactly like larvae—specifically, the coconut worm larvae (eaten live in Vietnam).

HORSERADISH: A member of the *Brassica* genus, along with mustard, broccoli, and rutabaga, horseradish root is a powerfully pungent root that is mainly used as a condiment. The easiest way to purchase it is pre-grated, salted, packed—sometimes with a bit of beet—in a jar.

LOTUS ROOT: The lotus root, part of the aquatic lotus flower plant, is an important food in many Asian countries, where it is commonly preserved as a pickle to accompany meals. It is also sliced and dried. Dried lotus root slices are often floated in soups and stews.

OCA: This small edible tuber hails from the Andes, where it is roasted and eaten with meat. It looks like a cross between a fingerling potato and an insect larva, though it tastes a bit like a potato.

PARSLEY ROOT: Looking very much like chubby parsnips, parsley roots are the sturdy roots of some types of parsley leaves. They taste a bit like a cross between celery and parsley and are popular in Holland, Germany, and Poland, where they are enjoyed boiled or roasted.

TARO: Starchy and bland, taro is sometimes called dasheen and is a popular and filling food throughout the West Indies, Africa, and Southeast Asia.

TIGER NUT: This small, sweet-tasting tuber is an important food in Africa—so important that Egyptians were often buried with these diminutive tubers. Through trade and migration, the tiger nut arrived in Spain, where tiger nut is known as *chufa* and is often blended into a sweet, milk-like drink.

YACON: Hailing from South America and looking very much like a russet potato, the yacon is a slightly sweet vegetable with a refreshing, almost jicama-like texture. It is lovely raw or roasted.

it, the sweeter it will be. With time, jicama's natural sugars turn to starch (though jicamas are not particularly sweet to start with).

USAGE: In my home, we use jicama sticks or planks as part of a veggie tray as dippers for salsa, hummus, and guacamole, and on sandwiches. They are terrific juiced or grated into a slaw or diced into prepared salsa. Not many people realize that jicama also takes well to cooking: I often throw a half cup of cubed jicama in soup or chili, and I like roasting it along with other roots.

BOTANICAL BACKGROUND: Jicamas are members of the *Pachyrhizus* genus, a family of legumes. Even though the tuberous root of the jicama plant is what we enjoy, the plant is related to lentils and other legumes.

HISTORY: Jicama hails from Mexico, where the Nahuatal word for the veggie is *xicamatl*. Spanish explorers and missionaries to Mexico and Central America so enjoyed jicama that they carried it with them into South America and the West Indies, where it quickly became an important food crop. Spaniards also took jicama with them to the Philippines, where it became a favorite snack food, as well an ingredient in local desserts, pickles, and entrees. The veggie quickly spread throughout Southeast Asia. Today, you'll find it on the menu in Thailand, Singapore, Indonesia, Malaysia, China, and Japan.

GROWING INFORMATION: Jicama does not like cold weather and needs about 9 months of frost-free days to grow. Seeds can be sown directly into moderate soil, in full sun. Be sure to have a stake or trellis handy: Jicama grows on vines that can reach 15 feet or more.

THINGS TO BE AWARE OF: The jicama plant has lovely, full leaves and seedpods with lima-like beans. Neither can be eaten, as they can cause respiratory distress and failure.

STEPHANIE'S FAVORITE USES: We eat jicama almost daily at my house. We like it shredded into slaws, cubed into salads, and chunked and roasted, but I think my favorite way to use it is as a dipper: We use it to scoop up salsa and guacamole.

JICAMA: DID YOU KNOW?

- Jicama was once cultivated for its seeds. The mature seeds of the jicama plant contain significant levels of rotenone, used in commercial insecticides.

- Jicama vines bear a white flower. Removing these flowers as buds is said to yield better root production.

- Most of the jicama found in North American and European markets is grown in Mexico and South America.

PARSNIP

NUTRITIONAL PROFILE PER SERVING
(1 CUP RAW; 133 G)

Calories: 99
Fiber: 7 g
Protein: 2 g
Vitamin C: 23 mg
Vitamin E: 2 mg
Vitamin K: 30 mcg
Copper: 0.8 mg
Folate: 89 mcg
Magnesium: 39 mg
Manganese: 0.7 mg
Omega-3 fatty acids: 4 mg
Pantothenic acid: 0.8 mg
Phosphorus: 95 mg
Potassium: 499 mg

ROLE IN SUPPORTING HEALTH

HELPS PREVENT LEUKEMIA: Parsnips are rich in several phytonutrients. One of these, called falcarinol, has been shown by researchers at Austria's Institut für Pharmazie der Universität Innsbruck to be a powerful chemopreventative with the ability to prevent and kill leukemia cells. Scientists isolated this compound in parsnips using nuclear magnetic resonance spectroscopy, mass spectrometry, and optical rotation data.

COMBATS OXIDATIVE STRESS: In simple terms, oxidative stress is a breakdown of the body's cells due to environmental factors or negative body actions (the stress-induced release of large amounts of cortisol, for instance). Falcarinol—which parsnips are rich in—has been found to help repair this oxidative stress in muscle tissue cells. Researchers at the University of Aarhus in Denmark took tissue samples of healthy human muscle fiber and subjected them to a range of damaging substances and processes. They found that tissue treated with falcarinol was less likely to be damaged or die than muscle tissue that was not treated with falcarinol.

GENERAL INFORMATION

PURCHASING: Look for firm, smooth roots that feel heavy for their size. Parsnips should be free of cuts, blemishes, and weepy spots, and they should not be withered.

STORAGE: Store unwashed parsnips in a storage bag and place in the produce drawer of your refrigerator. They should keep for up to 2 weeks.

USAGE: Parsnips are commonly added to soups and stews or tossed with other root veggies into a roasting pan. But they are also wonderful sliced into "coins" and pan-fried, braised, or boiled and mashed. They can also be enjoyed raw—juice them, shred them, slice them thin into salads, or enjoy them anywhere you'd usually use carrots.

BOTANICAL BACKGROUND: A member of the Apiaceae family, parsnips are related to carrots and parsley.

HISTORY: Parsnips have been used as food since before the Middle Ages and were an important food crop in Rome, where they were eaten as a vegetable and used as a sweetener (a role they played for centuries, until the mid-1500s, when inexpensive cane sugar from the New World began appearing in Europe).

GROWING INFORMATION: Parsnip seeds can be directly sown into well-tilled, well-drained soil during early spring. They enjoy sun or partial shade and a moderate amount of water.

THINGS TO BE AWARE OF: Parsnip leaves contain a sap that can cause photodermatitis, a discoloration of the skin that occurs when ultraviolet light interacts with this sap. For this reason, it's smart to wear gloves when harvesting parsnips.

STEPHANIE'S FAVORITE USES: Parsnips can be used almost anywhere that carrots are, meaning they are perfect in soups, stews, and baked goods. When I make homemade hash browns, I adore subbing half the potatoes with parsnips.

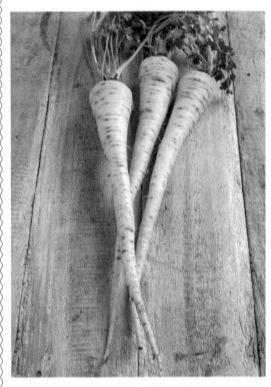

Beautiful parsnips are delicious in soups and stews.

POTATOES

NUTRITIONAL PROFILE PER SERVING

(1 CUP COOKED; 173 G)

GOLD

Calories: 132
Fiber: 4 g
Protein: 6 g
Vitamin C: 100 mg
Vitamin K: 5 mcg
Betaine: 0.3 mg
Choline: 33 mg
Copper: 0.3 mg
Folate: 47 mcg
Iron: 2 mg
Magnesium: 49 mg
Manganese: 0.3 mg
Niacin: 3 mg
Omega-3 fatty acids: 18 mg
Pantothenic acid: 0.6 mg
Phosphorus: 125 mg
Potassium: 620 mg
Thiamin: 0.1 mg

PURPLE

Calories: 132
Fiber: 2 g
Protein: 4 g
Vitamin A: 90 IU
Vitamin C: 900 mg
Vitamin K: 5 mcg
Beta-carotene: 15 mcg
Betaine: 0.3 mg
Choline: 33 mg
Copper: 0.3 mg
Folate: 47 mcg
Iron: 2 mg
Lutein: 60 mcg
Magnesium: 49 mg
Manganese: 0.3 mg
Niacin: 3 mg
Omega-3 fatty acids: 18 mg
Pantothenic acid: 0.6 mg
Phosphorus: 125 mg
Potassium: 510 mg
Thiamin: 0.1 mg

PINK/RED-FLESH

Calories: 154
Fiber: 3 g
Protein: 4 g
Vitamin B6: 0.4 mg
Vitamin C: 22 mg
Vitamin K: 5 mcg
Beta-carotene: 11 mcg
Betaine: 0.3 mg
Choline: 33 mg
Copper: 0.3 mg
Folate: 47 mcg
Iron: 2 mg
Lutein: 54 mcg
Magnesium: 49 mg
Manganese: 0.3 mg
Niacin: 3 mg
Omega-3 fatty acids: 18 mg
Pantothenic acid: 0.6 mg
Phosphorus: 125 mg
Potassium: 943 mg
Thiamin: 0.1 mg

ROLE IN SUPPORTING HEALTH

FIGHTS INFLAMMATION AND IMPROVES IMMUNE SYSTEM FUNCTION:

Researchers from Washington State University studied the effects of pigmented potatoes on inflammation and immune response in healthy adult males. Twelve men, aged 18 through 40, were given 150 grams of cooked white (russet), gold, or purple-flesh potatoes (PP) once a day for 6 weeks in a double-blind study. Blood was collected at the beginning and again at the end of the study and analyzed for total antioxidant capacity and DNA damage. Participants who received gold or purple potatoes daily had reduced DNA damage and inflammation and higher blood antioxidant levels than those who ate white potatoes daily.

LOWERS BLOOD PRESSURE:
In a new study conducted at the University of Pennsylvania, at Scranton, 18 patients who were primarily overweight or obese with high blood pressure ate six to eight purple potatoes (each about the size of a golf ball) with skins twice daily for a month. Scientists monitored the patients' blood pressure, both systolic (the first of the two numbers in a blood pressure reading) and diastolic. The average systolic blood pressure dropped by 3.5 percent and the diastolic decreased by 4.3 percent.

GENERAL INFORMATION

PURCHASING: Regardless of color or size, potatoes should be very firm with smooth skin and an absence of bruises, weepy spots, withering, or cuts. You'll easily find golden (Yukon) varieties at markets everywhere. Some of the better-stocked markets—and certainly a large farmer's market—may also carry some of the blue/purple- and pink-flesh varieties.

STORAGE: Store unwashed, uncut potatoes in a cool, dark place for up to 2 months. Make sure to store them away from onions, which let off a gas that can cause potatoes to spoil. And speaking of spoiling, be sure to remove any soft or visibly spoiled potatoes before storing them. One bad potato can affect the entire bunch.

USAGE: Potatoes are incredibly versatile. Boil them, mash them, steam them, bake them, roast them, puree them, fry them, sauté them, braise them. You can even grate raw potatoes to use as a cooling pack for sunburned or burned skin. Try it! (And while I'm not sure I'd recommend cooking and eating them after that, I would definitely compost the remains.)

BOTANICAL BACKGROUND: Potatoes—regardless of their color or size—are members of the Solanaceae, or nightshade, family. Other members of this family include eggplants, chiles, and tomatoes.

HISTORY: Though the potato is closely associated with Ireland, Idaho, and Northern Europe, this important food is actually from the Andes, a mountainous region of Peru. They were first "discovered" by Spaniards who were in South America for the Spanish conquest of the Inca Empire in the mid-sixteenth century. The Spanish called the vegetable *patata*, after the Quechua word *papa*, which the locals called it. It took Europeans several centuries to begin growing potatoes in large quantities, but once they did (during the late eighteenth century), the vegetable became very popular.

GROWING INFORMATION: Potatoes love cooler temperatures. Look for a location that gets full or partial sun. Soil should be well tilled, loose, enriched with manure, and well drained. In the spring, after the danger of the last frost has passed, you can plant seed potatoes about 4 inches deep with eyes up, about 1 foot apart. Water moderately as they grow. Harvest about 10 weeks later.

POTATOES: DID YOU KNOW?

- There are roughly 5,000 varieties of potatoes, 99 percent of which are descended from a single species.

- The global average for potato consumption is 33 kg—in some form or another— each year, though there are many countries where potato consumption is higher. The average yearly consumption by individuals in Belarus is 180 kg, while individuals of Kyrgyzstan consume an average of 140 kg a year.

- In the U.S., several days are claimed as "National Potato Day," including August 19th and March 31st.

- French fries were introduced to the U.S. when Thomas Jefferson served them in the White House during his presidency of 1801–1809.

- In 1853, railroad magnate Commodore Cornelius Vanderbilt was dining in a fashionable resort at Saratoga Springs, New York. An exacting man, Vanderbilt sent his potatoes back to the restaurant kitchen because he felt they were cut too thick. Chef George Crum, annoyed at Vanderbilt's request for thinner-sliced potatoes, cut a potato into paper-thin slices, fried them in hot oil, and salted and served them. Vanderbilt loved his "Saratoga Crunch Chips," and the potato chip was born.

THINGS TO BE AWARE OF: While many root vegetables have edible leaves, potatoes do not. The leaves are toxic and can cause gastric distress, headache, shock, and paralysis.

STEPHANIE'S FAVORITE USES: Every Sunday I boil 5 pounds of red, blue, or gold potatoes. The moment they go from firm to semi-firm, I remove them from the boiling water, cool them, and store them in the fridge. Through the week I dice them into salads, sauté them with chickpeas and spinach in homemade curry sauce, mash them, fry them, and more. I do not have any one favorite way to enjoy this lovely veggie!

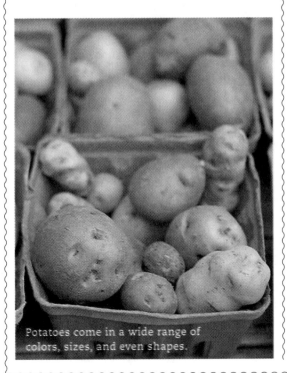

Potatoes come in a wide range of colors, sizes, and even shapes.

RADISH

NUTRITIONAL PROFILE PER SERVING (1 CUP RAW; 116 G)

Calories: 18
Fiber: 2 g
Protein: 0.8 g
Vitamin C: 18 g
Beta-carotene: 4.6 mcg
Betaine: 0.1 mg
Choline: 8 mg
Fluoride: 7 mcg
Folate: 29 mcg
Lutein: 12 mcg
Omega-3 fatty acids: 36 mg
Potassium: 270 mg
Phytosterols: 8 mg

ROLE IN SUPPORTING HEALTH

REDUCES HYPERTENSION: A team of researchers from Kookmin University in South Korea gave powdered radish leaves to hypertensive rats daily for 5 weeks. One group received 30 milligrams of powdered radish leaves per kilogram of body weight. Another group received 90 milligrams per kilogram of body weight. All animals had their blood pressure checked weekly. At the end of the study, researchers reported that both groups saw significant and similar reductions in their blood pressure (although they did not give the exact numbers).

PROTECTS THE LIVER: Eating radishes to improve liver health is a folk remedy in Japan, Korea, and China. Sulfurous chemicals in radishes help the free flow of bile. Bile carries toxins into the gallbladder then on into the small intestine, so they can be excreted. Radish is also said to reduce hardened deposits in the liver, as well as aid digestion. Research supports this. A study from the Dong Nam Institute of Radiological and Medical Sciences in Korea found that radish can help heal liver tissue that has been damaged by toxic medication, including chemotherapy drugs, and can also protect the liver from damage by medications used to treat symptoms but that are filtered by the liver.

OTHER LIVER PROTECTION: Radishes contain a special compound known as RsPHGPx, an antioxidant that helps protect the liver from damage while this important organ helps remove toxins from the body. These toxins include things we may ingest every day, including pain relievers, nicotine, insecticides, and carcinogenic molecules. Researchers from Tsinghua University in China looked at liver cells taken from mice. They found that, in vitro, the cells treated with this "radish compound"—RsPHGPx— were protected from damage when exposed to common toxins. Cells not treated with this compound became damaged.

REDUCES DAMAGING INFLAMMATION IN THE BODY: Inflammation has been named a culprit in diseases as far-ranging as cardiovascular disease, cancer, arthritis, and eczema. Radishes—and other members of the *Brassica* genus—contain a phytonutrient called indol-3-carbinol that has been shown in several studies to reduce inflammation. A study performed by researchers at Taipei Medical University in Taiwan looked at how this nutrient affected cells that were exposed to an agent that created inflammation. It was found that cells protected with indol-3-carbinol showed little inflammation compared with cells that were not treated with indol-3-carbinol.

GENERAL INFORMATION

PURCHASING: Look for firm roots that are heavy for their size. Avoid buying radishes that are bruised, withered, wrinkled, cut, or marked with weepy spots. If you buy radishes with the leaves (which can be juiced, sautéed, added to soup, or chopped into salads), choose those with bright, perky leaves devoid of slimy, wet, or yellow spots.

STORAGE: Store radishes unwashed in a storage bag or container in the vegetable drawer of your refrigerator for up to 5 days. If the leaves are intact, remove them and store them, unwashed, separately, in a storage bag in the vegetable drawer of your fridge.

USAGE: Radishes are typically eaten raw. They are often sliced onto buttered bread, enjoyed whole (maybe dipped into a well of salt), added to salads and slaws, or even juiced. But they can also be baked, roasted, sautéed, or boiled. The leaves are peppery and can be enjoyed raw in a salad, sautéed as a cooking green, or juiced.

BOTANICAL BACKGROUND: Radishes are another member of the large, fabulous *Brassica* clan, along with cabbage, kale, broccoli, and horseradish.

HISTORY: It is believed that radishes may have originated in ancient China and then moved throughout the continent to Europe and the Middle East. Radish is one of the oldest domesticated (and first recorded) vegetables; the name *radish* comes from the Latin word *radix*, meaning "root." It was the first nonnative plant introduced to North America, first planted on the continent in 1629 in what is now Massachusetts.

GROWING INFORMATION: Radishes are easy to grow, which is why so many schoolchildren plant them. They can be sown directly into well-tilled soil as soon as the threat of frost passes. Give them a spot that gets 5 or so hours a day of sun (but nothing too hot; radishes prefer cool and just-mild-enough temperatures), water in moderation, and snap your fingers! In just 21 days or so, you'll have your radishes. To harvest, grab hold of the stem near the ground and gently pull up.

THINGS TO BE AWARE OF: More than one bunch of radishes a day can cause digestive upset in those who have sensitive digestive tracts.

STEPHANIE'S FAVORITE USES: Each Sunday I roast a huge pan of roots. If I have radishes in the kitchen, they always end up in the roasting pan. I love roasted radishes! The heat softens their edge without removing it, and gives them a sophisticated, full-bodied flavor.

RADISHES: DID YOU KNOW?

- There are hundreds of varieties of radishes grown worldwide, reaching 2 percent of total global vegetable production.

- In Mexico, the annual Noche de Rabanos (Night of the Radishes) festival takes place 24 hours before Christmas Eve. Mexican sculptors create Nativity scenes using very large radishes.

- The strong, sharp flavor of radishes is caused by allyl isothiocyanates. These are oils that are also found in horseradish, mustard, and wasabi.

- In the U.S., most commercially grown radishes hail from California and Florida.

RUTABAGA

NUTRITIONAL PROFILE PER SERVING
(1 CUP COOKED; 140 G)

Calories: 50
Fiber: 4 g
Protein: 2 g
Vitamin B6: 0.1 mcg
Vitamin C: 35 mg
Beta-carotene 1.4 mcg
Calcium: 67 mg
Choline: 20 mg
Folate: 29 mcg
Magnesium: 33 mg
Manganese: 0.2 mg
Omega-3 fatty acids: 74 mg
Phosphorus: 82 mg
Potassium: 472 mg
Thiamin: 0.1 mg

ROLE IN SUPPORTING HEALTH

SHRINKS CANCEROUS TUMORS: Using cells from cancerous tumors found in hamsters, researchers from Jagiellonian University in Poland looked at the anticancer activity in rutabaga seeds and roots and the tender shoots of rutabaga plants, which are used as a salad microgreen. Their findings indicated that while shoots had the highest ability to shrink tumors and prevent new ones from forming, the roots and seeds were also potent in shrinking cancerous tumors.

PREVENTS CANCER: Researchers at University of Dundee in Scotland examined the role that glucosinolates played in preventing cancer. Glucosinolates are a compound of phytonutrients with strong antioxidant abilities. Rutabaga features this phytonutrient in generous amounts. After experimenting with how cancerous cells reacted to glucosinolates, researchers concluded that the phytonutrients work in two ways: They prevent a cell's DNA from becoming damaged and growing irregularly (which often happens when a cell "goes rogue" and becomes cancerous), and they shut down any cancerous growth that does occur.

IMPROVES DIGESTION: Rutabagas contain large amounts of dietary fiber, essential for maintaining a healthy digestive tract. Consuming fiber helps to decrease the risk of colon cancer, protects against type 2 diabetes, and lowers the risk of heart disease. Researchers at University of Washington in Seattle found that adding cruciferous vegetables—such as rutabaga—to test subjects' diets did more than just improve elimination. By weighing each subject, then adding 14 grams of *Brassica* vegetables per kilogram of each subject's body weight (so if a person weighed 70 kilograms— roughly 154 pounds—researchers would multiply 14 grams by 70 kilograms to give the test subject 98 grams, or about 3.5 ounces, of *Brassica* veggies per day), then taking stool samples at the beginning and end of the 21-day trial, researchers learned that *Brassica* vegetables actually helped build and improve colonies of helpful bacteria within the large intestine.

GENERAL INFORMATION

PURCHASING: Rutabagas are available in grocery stores and at farm stands. When you buy them in a grocery store, they will not have their greens and will be coated lightly with food-grade wax for protection. (You can peel this away with a vegetable peeler.) The best source of unwaxed rutabagas is a farmer. Look for heavy, unblemished roots. If you happen to purchase roots with their greens intact, these can be chopped and sautéed in the same way you'd cook turnip greens. They can also be juiced.

STORAGE: Store unwashed, unpeeled rutabagas for up to 6 weeks in a cool, dry place in your pantry or in your fridge's vegetable drawer. If the greens are intact, remove those and store them, unwashed, in a storage bag in the vegetable drawer of your refrigerator.

USAGE: Rutabagas can be roasted, baked, boiled, steamed, sautéed, pickled raw, shredded into slaws, or sliced thick into salads. Rutabagas can also be juiced.

BOTANICAL BACKGROUND: Rutabaga is part of the large *Brassica* genus, making it a cousin to broccoli, collards, cabbage, Brussels sprouts, radishes, and turnips. It is thought that rutabagas first appeared in the early seventeenth century as a cross between wild cabbage and domesticated turnips, perhaps in the Bohemia area of Europe, and found an adoring culinary following in Sweden, where it was known as *rutabaga*, or "thick root."

HISTORY: Because of its ability to grow in even the most marginal soils and climates, rutabagas were popular in the northern reaches of Europe where other vegetables did not easily grow. Several cultures relied on the rutabaga heavily, including Sweden, the British Isles, and Ireland. Throughout Celtic Europe, rutabagas were central to the celebration of the ancient Celtic festival Samhain (which today we associate with Halloween). Young boys ran through villages carrying jack-o'-lanterns, which were originally carved from rutabagas (or turnips). This tradition was based on the legend of a blacksmith named Jack, who, after playing several tricks on the devil, was sentenced to roam the earth for eternity. He found his way through darkness by hollowing out a rutabaga and using it as a lantern.

GROWING INFORMATION: When I was growing up, I remember old-timers saying that rutabagas should be sown 100 days before the first fall frost. Of course no one knows when the first fall frost will be, but you probably have an idea when the first frost was in years past. (This will be a different time, depending upon where you live.) Rutabagas do not love extreme heat—they are a cool-weather crop. Plant in partial shade or indirect sun—or full sun, if not too hot. The seeds can be sown directly into well-tilled soil, spacing plants about a foot apart. Harvesting rutabagas when they are small means a milder-tasting vegetable, but you can keep them in the ground until they grow large.

THINGS TO BE AWARE OF: Rutabagas can be difficult to cut. Remove any wax with a vegetable peeler, slice a sliver off so you have a flat side to rest the veggie on, then slice away. If you find the root is too dense to get your knife through, drop it into a pot of boiling water for a minute to slightly soften it. This is a trick I've had to use many times with large rutabagas!

STEPHANIE'S FAVORITE USES: Rutabaga is one of my favorite vegetables. I love it so many ways, but my favorite might just be cooked rutabaga cubes tossed with chopped bacon and a dressing made from bacon fat and vinegar.

SALSIFY AND SCORZONERA

NUTRITIONAL PROFILE PER SERVING
(1 CUP COOKED; 135 G)

Calories: 91
Fiber: 5 g
Protein: 4 g
Vitamin B6: 0.4 mg
Vitamin C: 70 mg
Calcium: 64 mg
Choline: 35 mg
Folate: 20 mcg
Magnesium: 25 mg
Manganese: 0.4 mg
Omega-3 fatty acids: 15 mg
Phosphorus: 75 mg
Potassium: 382 mg
Riboflavin: 0.3 mg
Thiamin: 0.1 mg

ROLE IN SUPPORTING HEALTH

REDUCES PAIN AND INFLAMMATION: Scorzonera are used traditionally in Turkey as a painkiller and anti-inflammatory remedy. Researchers from Gazi University in Turkey set out to study the painkilling, anti-inflammatory mechanisms of scorzonera. In what seems like a barbaric lab test, mice were treated with an irritant at their ears or hind paws, or they were given a chemical that would cause their abdomens to constrict.

Those affected mice that received extracts of scorzonera topically and orally showed a marked decrease in swelling and in the release of pain hormones.

HEALS WOUNDS AND REDUCES INFLAMMATION: In another scorzonera study performed at Gazi University, researchers took samples of human skin tissue from incisions. Some of the skin cells were treated in vitro with scorzonera extracts. Some were not. The tissue that was treated with scorzonera showed less inflammation. Furthermore, the incision scars that were directly treated with scorzonera extract healed faster and with fewer instances of infection than those that were not treated with scorzonera extract.

PREVENTS LIVER DAMAGE: Researchers at Lebanese American University in Lebanon looked at the power of salsify, a common Lebanese folk remedy for liver disease, liver dysfunction, and many types of cancer. Rats were divided into a control group and a group that was given chemically induced liver damage. One of the signs of liver damage is increased liver enzymes being released into the bloodstream. In the liver-damaged rats, these elevated levels of liver enzymes were brought to completely normal, healthy levels (matching the liver enzyme levels of the control rats) when they received a dose that correlated with 250 milligrams of salsify extract per kilogram of a rat's body weight.

GENERAL INFORMATION

PURCHASING: Salsify and scorzonera are actually two different vegetables that are related and used interchangeably. They are often mislabeled, one for the other, in markets—which is usually fine, as the taste, nutritional profile, uses, and storage are nearly identical. Both are long, cylindrical roots. Salsify has a brown or tan bark-like coating, and scorzonera (which are often labeled as "black salsify"), a black bark-like coating. Regardless of which you purchase, look for a firm, heavy root that is not withered and has no weepy spots or cuts.

STORAGE: Store roots unwashed in a storage bag in the produce drawer of your refrigerator, where they should keep for up to 3 weeks.

USAGE: Both salsify and scorzonera should be peeled (with a vegetable peeler) before use. Because the flesh of each discolors quickly, keep a bowl of acidulated water nearby to submerge freshly peeled roots or cut chunks. While both are fantastic shredded raw into slaws, they are commonly boiled and mashed, fried, or roasted.

BOTANICAL BACKGROUND: Both are members of the Asteraceae family and are related to dandelions.

THESE ARE BULBS, NOT ROOTS

There are very clear distinctions between types of veggies: Arugula is a salad green; haricot verts are a seedpod; celery is a stalk; fiddlehead ferns are a shoot, and on and on. But there is a family of confusing veggies that many people erroneously think are roots: bulbs. These vegetables are the underground or ground-level portion of a plant where the vegetable's nutrient reserves are stored. Here are some of the best-loved culinary bulbs:

FENNEL: Sometimes called anise, this Mediterranean veggie can be enjoyed raw, pickled, or cooked.

GARLIC: The ultimate kitchen bulb, garlic is one of the world's most popular ingredients, appreciated for its ability to flavor a wide range of savory foods. Used worldwide, garlic shows up in the cuisines of Asia, Europe, Africa, North America, and South America. Natural health aficionados love garlic for its high level of immune-boosting antioxidants.

KOHLRABI: A member of the *Brassica* genus, kohlrabi is a light green bulb (though the leaves can be sautéed and eaten as well). Kohlrabi is popular in Scandinavia, the Netherlands, Germany, and Eastern Europe, where it is roasted, chopped, and added to the soup pot, or grated and mixed with mayonnaise for a fresh salad.

LEEK: A member of the *Allium* genus, leeks are the ultimate soup veggie. They look a bit like scallions on steroids in that they have the same coloration and same shape (non-bulbing white root ends) as their smaller cousins, but they are much larger and more fibrous.

ONION: The *Allium* genus is an enormous one, with the largest branch being onions. White, yellow, red, sweet, pearl, spring, and so on— there are hundreds of types of onions. All add a pungent, savory bite to food when used raw or cooked.

RAMPS: A member of the wide-ranging *Allium* genus, Allium tricoccum is a North American species of wild onion. Sometimes called wild garlic or wild leeks, ramps are widespread across eastern Canada and the eastern United States. They appear in the early spring and enjoy a cult-like popularity among foodies who enjoy their strong aroma and sharp, aggressive taste.

SCALLIONS: These small, fresh-tasting onions are often known as green onions. Looking a bit like a diminutive leek, scallions don't form bulbs, so the white root end is the same width as the greens. They are usually enjoyed raw and add a bright note to salads and salsas.

SHALLOT: This diminutive member of the *Allium* genus has a mild, buttery taste and depth of flavor that makes it popular in the world of gourmet cooking, where it is used raw in vinaigrettes or cooked as a flavoring for other foods.

HISTORY: Salsify and scorzonera are thought to have originated in the Middle East and spread northward to Europe, where in the 1500s they were eaten to prevent and cure bubonic plague.

GROWING INFORMATION: Salsify and scorzonera are easily grown plants that love cooler weather. About a week or two before spring's last anticipated frost, find an area of rich soil situated in full sun and till well. Sow seeds about half an inch deep and a few inches apart. Roots are ready to harvest in 4–5 months.

THINGS TO BE AWARE OF: Both vegetables give off a milky, sticky, latex-like substance when cut. It is said that this sticky substance was chewed in pre–Industrial Age Europe as a type of early chewing gum. If you get this on your skin, simply rub it off with a bit of rubbing alcohol.

STEPHANIE'S FAVORITE USES: Both roots are delicious in a gratin, but I think I like them best cubed and added to my weekly pan of roasted root vegetables.

SUNCHOKE

NUTRITIONAL PROFILE PER SERVING (1 CUP COOKED; 150 G)

> Calories: 109
> Fiber: 3 g
> Protein: 3 g
> Vitamin B6: 0.1 mg
> Vitamin C: 6 mg
> Beta-carotene: 18 mcg
> Choline: 45 mg
> Copper: 0.2 mg
> Iron: 6 mg
> Magnesium: 26 mg
> Niacin: 2 mg
> Pantothenic acid: 0.6 mg
> Phosphorus: 117 mg
> Potassium: 643 mg
> Thiamin: 0.3 mg

ROLE IN SUPPORTING HEALTH

PREVENTS DIABETES AND FATTY LIVER DISEASE: To see if sunchokes could prevent diabetes in rodents, researchers at the University of Tokyo gave rats one of two diets: 60 percent fructose (to create a spike in blood sugar), or 60 percent fructose and 10 percent sunchoke powder. After 4 fructose-filled weeks, all of the rats' blood showed signs of diabetes, and all of their livers showed signs of fatty liver disease.

However, the rodents who received sunchoke powder displayed significantly milder cases.

MINIMIZES CANDIDA: Researchers from the College of Veterinary Medicine at Mississippi State University fed one group of mice a diet enriched with inulin and another group their standard mice food. After 6 weeks on these diets, both groups were inoculated with the fast-growing, virulent yeast *Candida albicans*. Seven days later, mice who received dietary inulin showed 50 percent fewer candida cells in their intestines than the mice who did not receive inulin.

SIGNIFICANTLY LOWERS DANGERS OF INTESTINAL INFECTIONS: In the same study, four other groups of mice—two eating an inulin-enriched diet for 6 weeks, the other two eating their standard mice food— were inoculated with salmonella or listeria. Among the salmonella-infected animals eating an inulin-enriched diet, 60 percent died; 80 percent of the no-inulin group died. In the listeria group, none of the inulin-eating mice died, while 30 percent of the no-inulin group died.

GENERAL INFORMATION

PURCHASING: Look for unblemished, firm roots without cuts.

STORAGE: Place sunchokes, unwashed, directly in the produce drawer of the refrigerator for up to a month.

USAGE: One of the most common ways to use sunchokes is to roast them. They are also lovely sliced, sautéed, fried, added to stir-fries, cubed into soups and stews, or mashed to replace half the potatoes in mashed potatoes.

BOTANICAL BACKGROUND: A member of the Asteraceae family, sunchokes are the root of a small sunflower called *Helianthus tuberosus*.

HISTORY: Europeans arriving in North America found people harvesting, storing, and eating sunchokes. The vegetable has a long storage life, which made it easy to send back to Europe, where it, in turn, was taken to North Africa.

GROWING INFORMATION: This sun-loving plant can be started directly in the garden 2 weeks after the last spring frost. Because sunchokes can become invasive, choose a roomy spot away from other vegetation and plant about 3 or 4 inches deep, a foot apart, in well-tilled soil. Water when the soil dries out and wait 4–5 months before harvesting.

THINGS TO BE AWARE OF: Sunchokes are delicious, but oh my, do they have the potential to cause gas and extreme, uncomfortable bloating. That special fiber, inulin, is to blame. Though they can be eaten raw, I'd advise against it for this reason; you'll be much more comfortable with cooked sunchokes. If you're worried, don't serve them at a dinner party, and stick to using them as one ingredient in a dish, instead of as a dish unto themselves.

STEPHANIE'S FAVORITE USES: Tossed in extra virgin olive oil, salt, and pepper and roasted whole.

THINGS TO DO WITH SUNCHOKES

- Peel and chunk sunchokes and add to your next pot of chicken soup.
- Use sunchokes as a substitute for water chestnuts in stir-fries.
- Deep-fry thin slices to make sunchoke chips.
- Add shredded raw sunchokes to latkes.
- Peel and slice sunchokes and then steam in a small amount of water with a squeeze of lemon until just fork-tender. Cool and add to salads and sandwiches.
- Cook and then puree sunchokes. Serve the puree as-is, or stir into mashed potatoes or cauliflower.
- Sauté sunchoke slices in olive oil with garlic and a squeeze of lemon and serve as a side dish.
- Use grated raw sunchokes as an extender in meatballs and meatloaf.

SWEET POTATO

NUTRITIONAL PROFILE PER SERVING
(1 CUP COOKED; 200 G)

Calories: 180
Fiber: 7 g
Protein: 4 g
Vitamin A: 38,433 IU
Vitamin B6: 0.6 mg
Vitamin C: 40 mg
Vitamin E: 1.4 mg
Vitamin K: 4.6 mcg
Alpha-carotene: 58 mcg
Beta-carotene: 23,000 mcg
Betaine: 69 mg
Calcium: 76 mg
Choline: 26 mg
Copper: 0.3 mg
Iron: 1.4 mg
Magnesium: 54 mg
Manganese: 1 mg
Niacin: 3 mg
Omega-3 fatty acids: 12 mg
Pantothenic acid: 1. 8 mg
Phosphorus: 108 mg
Potassium: 950 mg
Riboflavin: 0.2 mg
Thiamin: 0.2 mg

ROLE IN SUPPORTING HEALTH

HAS ANTICANCER EFFECTS: Researchers from the Chinese Academy of Agricultural Sciences in Beijing looked at cancerous colorectal cells in vitro. When treated with sweet potato protein, the cancer cells shrunk. Noncancerous colorectal cells, when treated with sweet potato protein, failed to become cancerous when introduced to human colorectal cancer cells, thus preventing cancer from forming.

KEEPS YOU REGULAR: A study by researchers from Nursing College of Soochow University in China looked at natural ways of treating a very common condition experienced by hospital patients: Constipation. Of 93 patients hospitalized with acute coronary disease, 44 were given a laxative and 49 were given servings of sweet potatoes with their meals, as well as acupressure massage and foot baths. According to researchers, the group getting the sweet potatoes experienced less incidence of further constipation, higher "subjective satisfaction with their bowel emptying during hospitalization," and less incidence of incomplete evacuation and colorectal obstruction.

MAY HELP WARD OFF LEUKEMIA: Researchers from China Medical University in Taiwan looked at the antiproliferative (cancer-preventing) effect of sweet potatoes on leukemia cells in vitro. Seventy-two hours after leukemia cells were treated with sweet potato extract, the cells showed no division or growth and in fact had shrunk.

GENERAL INFORMATION

PURCHASING: Look for firm roots that are heavy for their size. Avoid those with weepy spots, cuts or blemishes, or that are withered.

STORAGE: Store unwashed sweet potatoes in a cool, dark spot in your pantry, where they can stay for about 3 months.

USAGE: Baked, boiled, mashed, sliced, fried, braised, roasted—I even juice one every once in a while—sweet potatoes are delicious prepared all kinds of ways.

BOTANICAL BACKGROUND: Sweet potatoes are members of the Convolvulaceae family and are related to morning glories. Indeed, a sweet potato plant's flower looks very much like a charming white and fuchsia morning glory.

HISTORY: Sweet potatoes are thought to have originated in Central America, and there is evidence of indigenous people in North America eating sweet potatoes before the arrival of Europeans. Sweet potatoes have also been eaten in Polynesia, Hawaii, the Cook Islands, and New Zealand since 700 CE. It is thought that seafaring Polynesians visited Central America and traveled back home with them, stopping at various islands on the way, where they introduced locals to the delicious vegetable.

GROWING INFORMATION: Sweet potatoes do not like cold weather.

THINGS TO BE AWARE OF: Sweet potatoes and yams are actually two different veggies. Sweet potatoes are the native North American vegetable with the outrageously high nutrient content. Yams are a starchy, slightly sticky, white-flesh tuber from the Caribbean and other tropical and subtropical countries. The confusion around names may have begun when slaves in U.S. colonial times used the African word for yam—*nyami*—for the sweet potatoes they found growing in the Americas. The USDA requires that all "genuine" sweet potatoes be labeled as "sweet potatoes" and not "yams," but the confusion continues today.

STEPHANIE'S FAVORITE USES: I am fond of sweet potatoes baked in their jackets, split open, and dressed with black beans, salsa, and guacamole.

TURNIP

NUTRITIONAL PROFILE PER SERVING
(1 CUP, COOKED; 156 G)

> Calories: 36
> Fiber: 4 g
> Protein: 2 g
> Vitamin B6: 0.1 mg
> Vitamin C: 19 mg
> Choline: 15 mg
> Copper: 0.1 mg
> Folate: 14 mcg
> Manganese: 0.2 mg
> Omega-3 fatty acids: 50 mg
> Phytosterols: 9.1 mg
> Potassium: 276 mg

ROLE IN SUPPORTING HEALTH

KILLS CANCER CELLS (AND MORE): According to research done at Kyung Hee University in South Korea, a phytonutrient in turnips known as brassicaphenanthrene A has been shown to kill 86 percent of human breast cancer cells (MCF-7) in vitro after just 12 hours. Brassicaphenanthrene A also prevents up to 98 percent of oxidative damage to LDL cholesterol in vitro.

LOWERS BREAST CANCER RISK: A recent study from China of 6,000 women found that those who consumed 140 grams or more of *Brassica* genus vegetables—of which turnip is a member—each day had a 35 percent lower risk incidence of breast cancer than women who ate fewer or no servings of *Brassica* genus vegetables each day. Turnips and their cousins contain an antioxidant compound of phytonutrients called isothiocyanates, which researchers believe help prevent cells from turning cancerous, and they also kill cancer cells already existing in the body.

DECREASES PROSTATE CANCER RISK: Turnips contain a phytonutrient called diindolylmethane, an antioxidant nutrient that has been found to help prevent cancer and shrink cancerous tumors. In a study by researchers at Hallym University in South Korea, diindolylmethane was found to kill cancerous tumor cells in mice with prostate cancer. Recent studies on tissue samples from humans with prostate cancer show it can do the same thing for them.

REDUCES LUNG CANCER RISK: Several studies have found a correlation between high vegetable intake and lowered risk of lung cancer. Research from International Agency for Research on Cancer in Lyon, France, looked specifically at the effect *Brassica* vegetables have on individual's chance of developing lung cancer. Looking at the diets of 2,141 individuals with lung cancer and 2,168 individuals who did not have lung cancer, researchers noticed that those who did not have lung cancer ate cruciferous (another name for the *Brassica* genus) veggies every week. Researchers did not record how many servings of these vegetables the cancer-free test subjects ate, but they did note that those with lung cancer did not eat cruciferous vegetables weekly.

GENERAL INFORMATION

PURCHASING: Turnips can be purchased with their greens or without their greens. If I have the choice, I always go for turnips with their greens. The greens are delicious sautéed with garlic or chopped and used wherever you'd use spinach. Choosing turnips with their greens also gives you an indication of how fresh they are. Turnip roots should be firm and heavy without cuts, brown spots, or weepy spots.

STORAGE: Place unwashed turnips in a storage bag in your refrigerator's vegetable drawer. If the turnips have greens, remove them and store them (also unwashed) in a separate bag in the vegetable drawer. Roots can keep for up to 2 weeks; greens should be used within 3 days. To freeze roots or greens, clean and drop them into a large pot of salted boiling water. Boil them just until barely soft, then quickly remove and run them under cold water to stop the cooking process. Allow them to drain, then place them in a freezer container and stash in the freezer, where they can stay for up to 3 months.

USAGE: Turnip roots can be shredded or sliced thin and enjoyed raw. They can be juiced. But most of us are most familiar with turnips that are boiled, mashed, baked, roasted, sautéed, braised, or added to stews and soups. The greens are best chopped and sautéed or added to recipes where you'd use spinach, chard, collards, or other cooking greens.

BOTANICAL BACKGROUND: A member of the *Brassica* genus, the turnip's famous cousins include cabbage, collards, broccoli, Brussels sprouts, kohlrabi, and rutabaga.

HISTORY: It's unknown when turnips were first domesticated; they were already a well-established food in Greece and Rome well before the Common Era. Pliny the Elder writes that he considered the turnip one of the most important vegetables of his day, stating, "it should be spoken of immediately after corn, or the bean, at all events; for next to these two productions, there is no plant that is of more extensive use." The root has been—and continues to be—eaten throughout Europe, Northern Asia, and North America by both humans and livestock.

GROWING INFORMATION: Turnips are a cool-weather vegetable that can be sown directly in a garden in early to mid spring for a late spring harvest, or late summer to early fall for a late fall harvest. Turnip plants prefer partial shade or shade, mild weather, and well-drained soil; the tiny seeds can be sown directly in the garden.

THINGS TO BE AWARE OF: An interesting survey of 2,000 people performed by the British food delivery company Just Eat found that 88 percent of individuals injure themselves in the kitchen, and that 39 percent of those cases were because of a difficult-to-cut vegetable. According to the survey, turnips rank fourth among accident-inducing veggies. Why? Because people do not know how to cut them: Slicing a sliver from one side of the turnip will help it lie flat so you can keep your fingers out of the knife's way while slicing.

STEPHANIE'S FAVORITE USES: I always add cubed turnips to chicken soup.

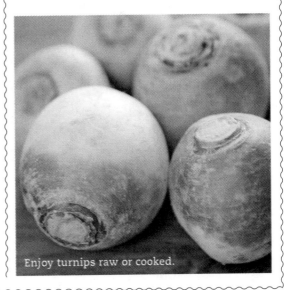
Enjoy turnips raw or cooked.

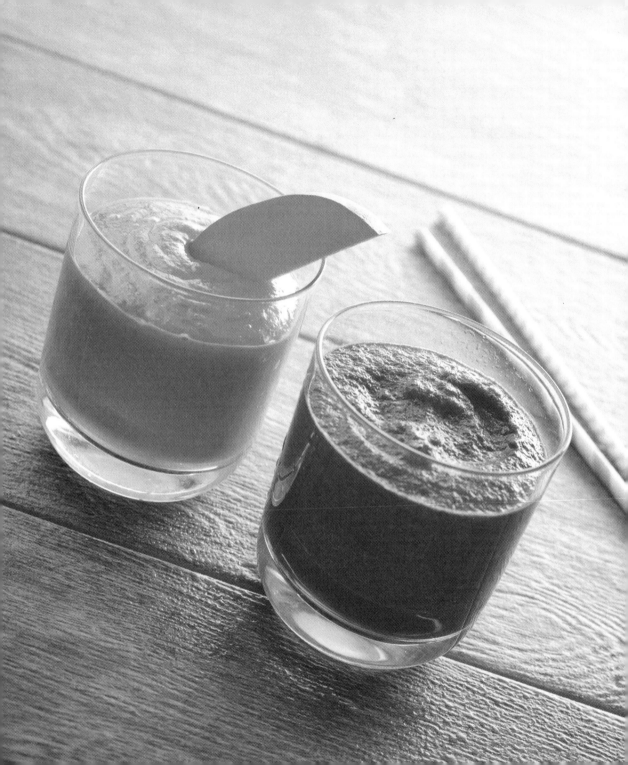

CHAPTER 2

DRINKS

Root veggies and beverages—not two things you'd expect in the same sentence, or in the same glass. But I'm here to tell you that roots have a long beverage-worthy history. Perhaps the most obvious recipes are teas. Medicinal and culinary teas made from burdock or salsify have been used as liver strengtheners and detoxifying concoctions for centuries. But root veggies also juice beautifully (my favorite is beet-red carrot juice with lemon) and can even be chunked and tossed into a blender as part of a satisfying smoothie. Keep reading for many more ideas!

HOT DRINKS

BEETROOT LATTE

MAKES 2 SERVINGS

Yes—I know: This one does sound odd. But no, I did not make this up to impress (or shock) you. Beetroot lattes (sometimes called red velvet lattes) are popular in Australia and the U.K. Try this recipe and you'll see why!

NOTE: You'll need a juicer for this one.

1 *cup milk of choice (coconut, almond, dairy, etc.)*

1 *large beet*

1 *small carrot*

½ *inch fresh ginger root*

1 *cup strong hot coffee*

Optional garnish: Sprinkle of cinnamon

1. In a pot over low heat, warm the milk.

2. While the milk warms, juice the beet, carrot, and ginger.

3. Add the fresh-pressed vegetable juice and hot coffee to the milk and stir to combine.

4. Pour the drink into two cups and, if desired, dust with ground cinnamon.

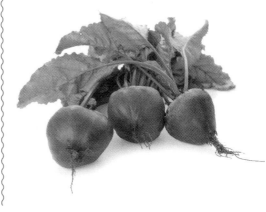

OPPOSITE: **Carrot-Mango Lassi (page 45) and Red Smoothie (page 46)**

BURDOCK TEA

MAKES 2 SERVINGS

Burdock tea is a time-honored diuretic and detoxification remedy used to stimulate bile production, reduce excessive levels of uric acid in the blood, and regenerate cells of the liver. I love this to reduce bloating, and my son finds it great for reducing the severity of his eczema (he drinks one cup of it and lets the other cup cool, which he then sponges directly on affected areas).

1   *fresh burdock root*

3   *cups water*

1. Using a vegetable brush, clean the burdock root. Then chop it coarsely.

2. Add the root to a pot and cover with the water.

3. Bring it to a boil, then lower the heat and simmer for 30 minutes.

4. Turn the heat off, cover the pot, and allow the root to steep for an additional 20 minutes.

5. Strain out the burdock pieces (I like to add the cooked burdock to soups and grain dishes) and pour the liquid into serving cups.

NOTE: Feel free to let this cool and drink it as an iced tea, or blend it with other tea flavors.

HOMEMADE BURDOCK AND DANDELION SODA

MAKES ABOUT 10 SERVINGS

Burdock and dandelion soda is a popular drink in Ireland, Scotland, Wales, and England, where some form of the beverage has been enjoyed since the Middle Ages, and is based on a recipe used by St. Thomas Aquinas. This version, while not exactly a health drink, is a fun way to use the root.

2   *teaspoons burdock root, chopped*

1   *teaspoon dandelion root, chopped*

1   *teaspoon ginger root, finely chopped*

1   *star anise*

1   *teaspoon lemon juice*

2½ *cups water*

1   *cup white sugar*

1. Add all ingredients to a saucepan over medium-high heat. Bring to a boil.

2. Lower heat to medium and allow to simmer for 20 minutes.

3. Allow mixture to cool.

4. Pour through a colander or strainer and place in a sealable bottle or container. Refrigerate and use within two weeks.

5. To make soda, add 2 or 3 tablespoons of syrup to 6–8 ounces of sparkling water. May also be used with vodka for an alcoholic drink.

SALSIFY TEA

MAKES 2 SERVINGS

Salsify contains high amounts of inulin, a prebiotic fiber that increases the growth of helpful bacteria, called bifidobacteria, in your gut. In turn, this boosts your immune system, helps your body absorb nutrients, and can even reduce carcinogens in your intestines. All good things!

1   *fresh salsify root or black salsify root*

3   *cups water*

1. Using a vegetable brush, clean the salsify root. Then chop it coarsely.

2. Add the root to a pot and cover with the water.

3. Bring it to a boil, then lower the heat and simmer for 30 minutes.

4. Turn the heat off, cover the pot, and allow the root to steep for an additional 20 minutes.

5. Strain out the salsify pieces (I like to add the cooked salsify to casseroles and soups) and pour the liquid into serving cups.

NOTE: Feel free to let this cool and drink as an iced tea, or blend it with other tea flavors.

SMOOTHIES AND OTHER BLENDER DRINKS

BEET-AND-CELERIAC-GREENS SMOOTHIE

MAKES 2 (OR MORE) SERVINGS

If you've ever wondered what to do with the greens from your roots, I urge you to give this a try. I like it best with beet and celeriac greens, but feel free to use a small amount of carrot, radish, or other root greens (yes, they are edible, but so strong, they may overpower your drink, so use sparingly). See "Root Greens and Their Uses" (page 44) for more on which greens are safe (and tasty) to consume.

1   *bunch of fresh beet greens, excluding stalks, washed and chopped*

1   *bunch of fresh celeriac greens, including stalks, washed and chopped*

½   *cup fresh or frozen fruit of your choice (I like frozen mango or pineapple)*

½   *Granny Smith apple, peeled and chopped*

1   *lime or lemon, peeled and chopped*

1   *14-ounce can coconut milk*

A few ice cubes (optional)

Add all ingredients to a blender and process until smooth. Add water if you'd like a thinner consistency.

ROOT GREENS AND THEIR USES

BEET: Kin of chard (in Australia, chard is called silverbeet), beet greens are lovely sautéed in your favorite oil and eaten as a cooked green. They also do well in the juicer, stems and all. Nutrients include vitamins C and K.

BURDOCK: The leaves are tough and chewy, but if harvested when the plant is young, they are soft, with an artichoke-like taste (which has made them a delicacy in Japan).

CARROT: Herbal in taste, with a chewy texture, antioxidant-rich carrot greens are great thrown in the stockpot or added—in small amounts—to grain or bean dishes (à la parsley). Despite Internet rumors, they are not poisonous and are, in fact, a market veggie in Europe.

CASSAVA: *Do not eat!* Cassava leaves contain high amounts of cyanogenic glucosides, which are toxic to humans and animals.

CELERIAC: Have you ever chopped the leaves of celery stalks into a salad? Then you know what celeriac greens taste like. Rich in potassium, they make a great garnish for potato or grain dishes and can be used in place of celery in potato or egg salad—or even soups.

JICAMA: You may never see a jicama sold with its leaves. That's because the leaves contain a neurotoxin that is poisonous to humans.

PARSNIP: *Avoid.* The juice from the leaves creates a strong skin reaction.

POTATO: *Avoid* the leaves, which are poisonous. They contain a glycoalkaloid toxin, which causes weakness, confusion, coma, and then death.

RADISH: If you like arugula, you'll love radish greens. These peppery, bitter, chlorophyll-rich greens are fun to add to salads and (in small amounts) green juice and smoothies. But I like them best in potato and leek soup or chopped and added to meatballs.

RUTABAGA: The leaves are edible, but go for the young ones. The older ones are tough and chewy (which, come to think of it, makes them fine for juicing). When cooked, the young ones taste a bit like collards.

SALSIFY: If you get salsify leaves while they are still tender, they make a peppery addition to salads or can be tossed into soups and stir-fries, or juiced.

SWEET POTATO: Soft, with a flavor akin to chard (but much milder), sweet potato greens are delicious and rich in fiber and vitamin C.

SUNCHOKE: As a member of the sunflower family, sunchokes have large, tough, almost sandpapery leaves that do not taste pleasant.

TURNIP: Bitter and wonderful, turnip greens are a pot green, much like collards or kale. Cooked chopped turnip greens are terrific in soups and stews and wonderful in a frittata, where they add color, fiber, and vitamins A, C, and K.

CARROT-MANGO LASSI

MAKES 1–2 SERVINGS

Ask any of my kids their favorite thing about going out for Indian food and they'll say the mango lassis. This homemade version is just as delicious as what you get at the local curry shop, but has the added health benefits of carrots (beta-carotene, antioxidants, fiber) and coconut milk. You're going to love this one!

- 2 *medium carrots, cleaned and roughly chopped*
- 1 *cup mango (fresh or frozen)*
- ½ *cup coconut milk*
- 3 *tablespoons coconut nectar or honey*
- 1–2 *tablespoons fresh lime juice*
- *A few ice cubes (optional)*

Add all ingredients to a blender and process until smooth. Add water if you'd like a thinner consistency.

PARSNIP SMOOTHIE

MAKES 1–2 SERVINGS

Parsnips are funny in a "taste like dirt" kind of way, which is why I did not want to try this smoothie when a cooking instructor friend first made it for me. I am nothing if not intrepid, though, so try it I did. And liked it! I bet you will, too.

- 2 *medium parsnips, washed*
- ½ *cup frozen pineapple*
- ½ *cup frozen mango*
- 1 *cup coconut milk*
- 1 *tablespoon chia seeds*

Add all ingredients to a blender and process until smooth. Add water if you'd like a thinner consistency.

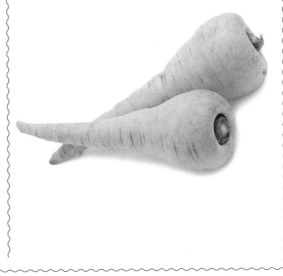

SWEET POTATO SMOOTHIE

MAKES 1–2 SERVINGS

My kids love this one. It is sweet and (thanks to the lemon or lime) tangy. It is lovely in cool weather and filling enough to enjoy as a snack. If you'd like to enjoy this for breakfast, add a tablespoon or two of nut butter for protein.

- 1 cup cooked sweet potato or puree (cooked without salt or spices)
- 1 14-ounce can coconut milk
- ½-inch piece fresh ginger
- ¾ cup lemon or lime juice
- Dash of cinnamon
- Dash of nutmeg or allspice
- A few ice cubes (optional)

Add all ingredients to a blender and process until smooth. Add water if you'd like a thinner consistency.

RED SMOOTHIE

MAKES 1–2 SERVINGS

This pretty drink is deeply nutritious and delicious. This will also be an easier drink for your kids to accept than a green smoothie. Feel free to play with the fruit, adding, subtracting, or changing as desired.

- 1 small red beet, peeled
- ½ navel orange, peeled
- 1 handful frozen berries
- 1 handful fresh or frozen kale
- ¼ cup frozen pineapple (optional)
- 1 cup cold water

Add all ingredients to a blender and process until smooth. Add more water if you'd like a thinner consistency.

JUICES

RADISH JICAMA JUICE

MAKES 1 SERVING

Thanks to the diuretic nature of radish and jicama, this cleansing juice is a great choice for when you feel bloated and lethargic. Be sure to wash all produce before juicing.

- 1 *large radish*
- 1 *large tart apple, such as Granny Smith*
- ½ *jicama*
- 1 *lemon, peeled*
- 1 *handful cilantro*

1. Cut all ingredients, if necessary, to fit into the feed tube of a juicer.

2. Feed all ingredients, in the order listed, through the feed tube.

3. Enjoy immediately.

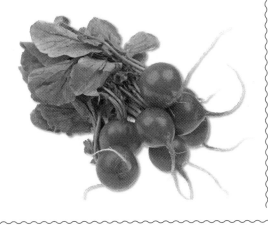

RUTABAGA JUICE COCKTAIL

MAKES 1 SERVING

Rutabaga has a strong, sharp taste—one that I crave. I even like rutabaga juice. If it sounds weird to you, I encourage you to try this. It is refreshing, energizing, and high in vitamins C and B complex, plus it helps strengthen the liver.

- 1 *cup chopped raw rutabaga*
- 1 *lemon, peeled*
- 1 *tart apple, such as a Granny Smith*
- 1 *celery stalk*
- 1 *sprig parsley*

1. Cut all ingredients, if necessary, to fit into the feed tube of a juicer.

2. Feed all ingredients, in the order listed, through the feed tube.

3. Enjoy immediately.

CELERIAC JUICE

MAKES 1 SERVING

Refreshing and thirst quenching, this is a great juice to enjoy on a sweaty day or after working out. Celeriac contains generous amounts of sodium, potassium, magnesium, and other electrolytes.

1   cup peeled, chopped celeriac root

1   Asian pear, chopped

½   lemon, peeled

1. Cut all ingredients, if necessary, to fit into the feed tube of a juicer.

2. Feed all ingredients, in the order listed, through the feed tube.

3. Enjoy immediately.

PPL JUICE

MAKES 1–2 SERVINGS

This sweet drink has an autumnal quality thanks to the parsnips and pears, that I always associate with fall. You will enjoy this grounding drink.

2   parsnips, washed and roughly chopped

2   pears, washed and quartered

2   lemons or limes, peeled and quartered

1. Cut all ingredients, if necessary, to fit into the feed tube of a juicer.

2. Feed all ingredients, in the order listed, through the feed tube.

3. Enjoy immediately. Or, for something different, warm the juice in a saucepan and enjoy hot.

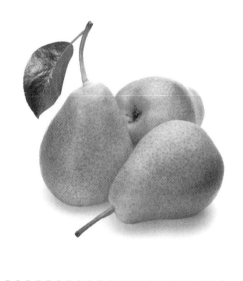

VEGGIE FUSION JUICE

MAKES 1–2 SERVINGS

This mixed-veggie beverage is a fantastic way to start the day. It's also a terrific mid-afternoon pick-me-up. Feel free to use different veggies or herbs if you'd like.

5   *carrots, washed and roughly chopped*

3   *leaves spinach*

4   *leaves romaine lettuce*

1   *small turnip*

1   *stalk celery*

Small handful parsley or dill or cilantro

1   *orange, peeled and quartered*

1. Cut all ingredients, if necessary, to fit into the feed tube of a juicer

2. Feed all ingredients, in the order listed, through the feed tube.

3. Enjoy immediately.

CARROT-ORANGE JUICE

MAKES 1–2 SERVINGS

This is a classic veggie-fruit juice, one of the first available when I was a young adult. It offers up large amounts of beta-carotene and vitamin C and a host of antioxidants. Plus, almost everyone likes it. I like to add half a lemon or lime to the mix.

3   *medium carrots, washed and roughly chopped*

2   *medium oranges, peeled and quartered*

1. Cut all ingredients, if necessary, to fit into the feed tube of a juicer.

2. Feed all ingredients, in the order listed, through the feed tube.

3. Enjoy immediately.

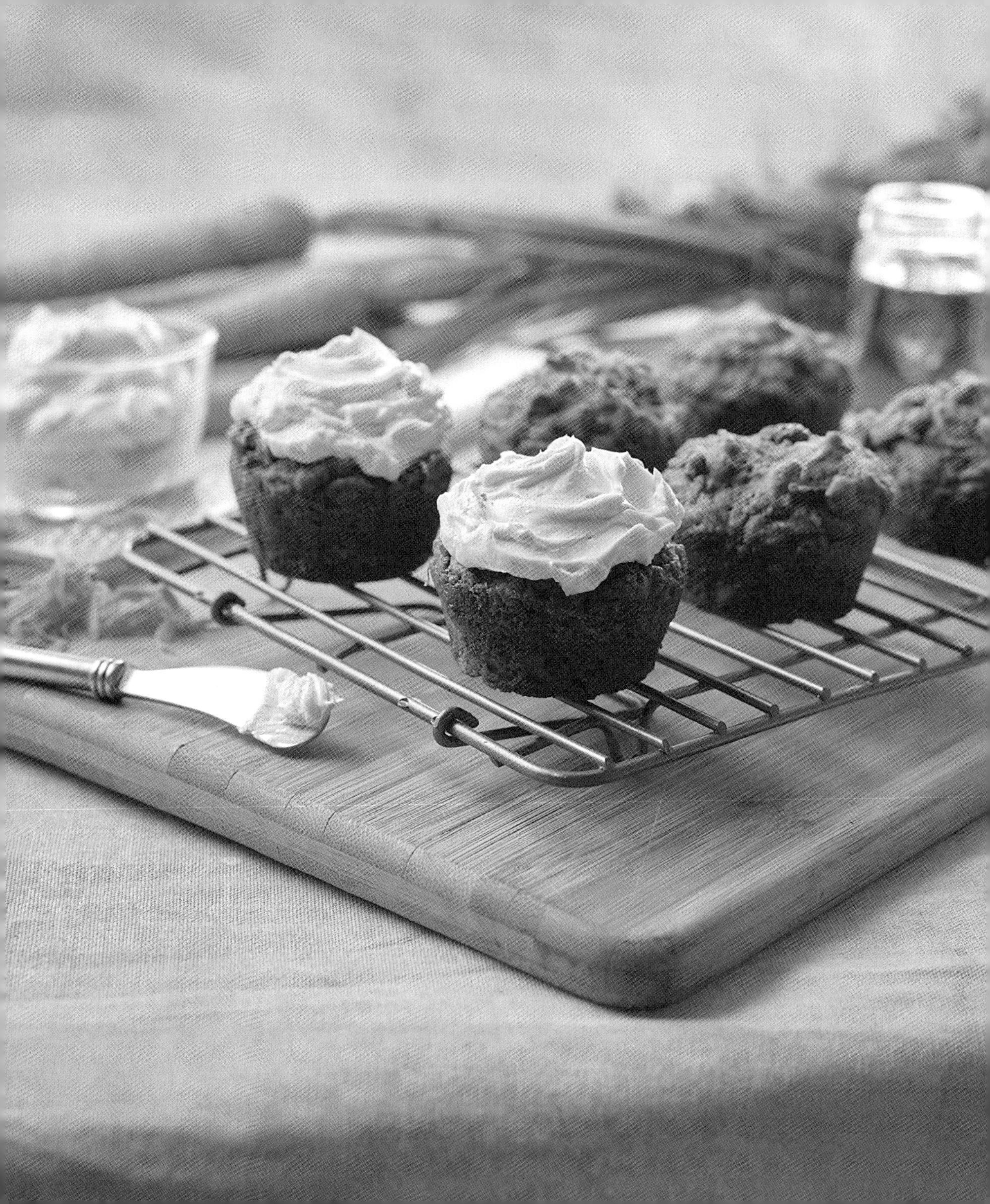

CHAPTER 3

BREAKFAST

Roots are a natural breakfast ingredient, at least in my world. I love Glory Muffins with grated parsnip and carrots, beet juice, sautéed root-veggie hash with eggs, and more. Root veggies not only provide large amounts of nourishing vitamins, minerals, and fiber, but they also fill us up and leave us feeling grounded and ready to face the day.

BAKED GOODS

BEET NO-WHEAT SCONES

MAKES ABOUT 8

Because I feel better without gluten, I am always looking for tasty recipes that use alternative flours. This superfood scone recipe—featuring coconut milk, among other good things—fits the bill. And that it contains grated beets? So much the better! **NOTE:** This isn't the easiest dough to work with—it's sticky! Resist the temptation to use a rolling pin here and instead pat it out by hand on a floured surface (use the same gluten-free flour that you used in the recipe).

1¾ cups gluten-free multipurpose flour

⅓ cup sugar

2 teaspoons baking powder

½ teaspoon xanthan gum

½ teaspoon salt

½ cup (1 stick) cold butter or solid coconut oil

¾ cup grated raw beet or other grated root veggie

2 large eggs

⅓ cup cold coconut milk (do not use "lite")

1 teaspoon gluten-free vanilla extract

1. Preheat the oven to 400°F.

2. Grease a large baking sheet (or line with parchment).

3. Whisk together the gluten-free flour, sugar, baking powder, xanthan gum, and salt.

4. Using a pastry cutter or a fork, work in the cold butter until the mixture is crumbly with pea-size bits of butter remaining.

5. Gently mix in the grated beets.

6. In another bowl, whisk together the eggs, milk, and vanilla. Add to the dry ingredients, gently folding in until everything is blended. The dough will be sticky.

OPPOSITE: **Carrot Cake Muffins (page 52)**

7. Turn the dough out onto a surface floured with gluten-free flour and pat out to about 1 inch thick.

8. Use a biscuit cutter to cut into circles, or cut the dough into triangles. Place the pieces on the prepared pan.

9. Place the baking sheet, uncovered, in the freezer for 15 minutes to firm up the unbaked scones. Bake for 15–20 minutes, or until golden brown. Remove from the oven and let rest for 5 minutes before serving.

CARROT CAKE MUFFINS

MAKES 18 MUFFINS

Muffins and root veggies are longtime friends. Make this recipe as written with grated carrots, or try sweet potatoes, parsnips, beets, or a combination of the three. Also feel free to substitute a cup of carrot, sweet potato, or parsnip puree for the applesauce. Enjoy! **NOTE:** This recipe makes about 18 muffins; you can purchase 18-cup muffin tins.

- 2 cups spelt or white wheat flour
- 2 teaspoons baking soda
- 1 teaspoon ground cinnamon
- ¼ teaspoon ground nutmeg
- 1 teaspoon salt
- 3 large carrots, shredded (about 2 cups)
- ⅓ cup chopped walnuts or pecans
- 1 cup thick applesauce (or pureed sweet potato, pumpkin puree, or mashed banana)
- ¼ cup maple syrup, amber or dark
- 2 large eggs
- 1 teaspoon vanilla
- ¼ cup liquid coconut oil

1. Preheat the oven to 350°F.

2. Prepare a muffin tin with paper cups. Set aside.

3. In a large mixing bowl, combine the flour, baking soda, cinnamon, nutmeg, salt, carrots, and walnuts until well mixed. Set aside.

4. In a small mixing bowl, combine the applesauce, maple syrup, eggs, vanilla, and coconut oil. Stir until smooth.

5. Add the applesauce mixture to the flour mixture and stir only to combine. A few unblended lumps of flour are fine. Too much mixing makes a tough muffin!

6. Spoon the mixture into the prepared muffin cups, filling the cups about halfway.

7. Bake for 15–20 minutes, or until the tops begin to crack and a toothpick inserted into the center comes out clean.

8. Remove from the oven and let cool completely on a baking rack.

GLORY MUFFINS

MAKES 18 MUFFINS

Parsnips were once a popular ingredient in all kinds of baked goods. I resurrect that nutritious tradition with this scrumptious muffin. If you don't have parsnips, carrots or sweet potatoes make a fine substitute. **NOTE:** This recipe makes about 18 muffins; you can purchase 18-cup muffin tins.

1   *cup pecans*

3   *parsnips, peeled and grated (about 2 cups)*

1   *large apple, peeled, cored, and grated*

1   *teaspoon lemon zest*

2   *cups spelt or white wheat flour*

¾   *cup raw (turbinado) sugar*

¾   *teaspoon baking soda*

1½ *teaspoons baking powder*

½   *teaspoon salt*

1   *teaspoon ground ginger*

½   *teaspoon grated nutmeg*

1½ *teaspoons ground cinnamon*

½   *cup dried unsweetened cranberries (or use ¾ cup fresh or frozen cranberries)*

2   *large eggs*

¾   *cup liquid coconut oil*

½   *cup coconut milk*

1½ *teaspoons pure vanilla extract*

1. Preheat the oven to 350°F.

2. Prepare a muffin tin with paper cups. Set aside.

3. Toast the pecans about 10 minutes, or until lightly browned and fragrant. Let cool and then chop coarsely.

4. Combine the parsnips, apple, and lemon zest in a large bowl and set aside.

5. In a second large bowl, whisk together the flour, sugar, baking soda, baking powder, salt, ginger, nutmeg, and cinnamon. Stir in the pecans and dried cranberries. Set aside.

6. In a third bowl, whisk together the eggs, oil, coconut milk, and vanilla.

7. Fold the egg mixture and the parsnip mixture into the flour mixture, stirring just until moistened and combined. A few unblended lumps of flour are fine. Too much mixing makes a tough muffin!

8. Spoon the mixture into the prepared muffin cups, filling the cups about halfway.

9. Bake about 20 minutes, or until muffins are a deep golden brown and a toothpick inserted in the center of a muffin comes out clean.

10. Remove from the oven and let cool completely on a baking rack.

MEXICALI RUTABAGA MUFFINS

MAKES 12 MUFFINS

Most of us think of muffins as sweet treats, but muffins can be savory as well. These yummy superfood muffins are delicious as an accompaniment to soup, stews, and (my favorite) chili, or as a nutritious snack.

1¼ cups spelt or white wheat flour

½ cup buckwheat flour

2 teaspoons baking powder

½ teaspoon salt

¼ teaspoon freshly ground black pepper

1 scallion, including part of the green, minced

2 tablespoons cilantro leaves, finely chopped

1 teaspoon freshly ground coriander seeds

2 large eggs

1 teaspoon honey

1½ cups rutabaga, peeled and finely shredded

1 red pepper, roasted, peeled and diced*

1 cup coconut milk

½ cup extra virgin olive oil (or liquid coconut oil or avocado oil)

*To roast bell peppers, grill or broil the peppers, turning regularly, until the skin blackens and begins to peel. Place into a paper or plastic bag and seal; the steam will help separate the skin. When they are cool enough to handle, they can be removed from the bag. The skin should peel off easily.

1. Preheat the oven to 400°F.

2. Prepare a muffin tin with paper cups. Set aside.

3. In a bowl, stir together the two flours, baking powder, salt, ground black pepper, scallion, cilantro, and coriander.

4. In a separate large bowl, beat the eggs until blended. Add the honey, rutabaga, red pepper, milk, and oil. Mix until well blended.

5. Gently fold the flour mixture into the egg mixture and mix only until just moistened. A few unblended lumps of flour are fine. Too much mixing makes a tough muffin!

6. Spoon the batter into the prepared muffin cups.

7. Bake for 15–18 minutes, or until a toothpick inserted in the center comes out just a little moist. Do not overbake them.

8. Remove the muffins from the oven and let cool completely on a baking rack.

9. These muffins can be stored for up to 2 days in an airtight plastic container.

ROOTY BREAKFAST CAKE

MAKES 8 SERVINGS

I have to admit that we don't serve a lot of cake in our home: Too much sugar, not enough nutrition, blah, blah, blah. This one, however, I make an exception for. The grated root veggies provide antioxidants and fiber, while the almond flour offers up protein. The coconut cream gives us a nice dose of immune-boosting lauric acid and heart-supportive medium chain fatty acids.

3 cups grated carrots or parsnips (or a combination), divided

1¾ cups almond flour, divided

1¼ cups spelt or white wheat flour, divided

Dash of nutmeg

½ cup liquid coconut oil, divided, plus more for the pan

1 cup raw sugar (such as turbinado or Sucanat), divided

1½ teaspoons baking powder

½ teaspoon baking soda

½ teaspoon salt

½ cup coconut cream

1 teaspoon pure vanilla extract

3 large eggs

1. Preheat the oven to 350°F.

2. Oil an 8-inch round or square pan and line the bottom with parchment paper.

3. In a medium bowl, make the crumb topping by combining 1 cup carrots, ¼ cup almond flour, ¼ cup spelt flour, nutmeg, ¼ cup sugar, and 1 tablespoon oil. Set aside.

4. In a large bowl, whisk together the remaining 1½ cups almond flour, remaining 1 cup spelt flour, baking powder, baking soda, and salt.

5. In a second large bowl, whisk together the coconut cream, vanilla, eggs, remaining ¾ cup sugar, and remaining 7 tablespoons of oil.

6. Add the flour mixture to the coconut cream mixture and whisk again until incorporated. Fold in the remaining 2 cups of carrots.

7. Transfer the batter to the prepared pan and scatter the crumb topping on top. Bake until the cake springs back in the middle when pressed and is deep golden brown, 50–60 minutes.

8. Set aside to let cool, then transfer to a plate, discarding parchment paper. Cut into squares or wedges and serve.

WAFFLES AND GRIDDLE CAKES

CARROT CAKE WAFFLES

MAKES ABOUT 6 SERVINGS

Do you like carrot cake? Then you'll love these waffles. They are like eating cake for breakfast. You can make them gluten-free by using your favorite gluten-free all-purpose flour mix.

1½ cups whole-wheat pastry flour

3 tablespoons coconut sugar, raw sugar, or brown sugar

1½ teaspoons baking powder

1 teaspoon ground cinnamon or pumpkin pie spice mix

½ teaspoon baking soda

¼ teaspoon salt

2 large eggs

1 cup coconut milk (do not use "lite") or buttermilk

2 tablespoons liquid coconut oil

¾ cup grated carrots

1. Lightly coat a waffle iron with cooking spray, and preheat to 200°F.

2. In a large bowl, whisk together the flour, sugar, baking powder, cinnamon, baking soda, and salt.

3. In a separate bowl, whisk together the eggs, coconut milk, and coconut oil until well blended.

4. Pour the egg mixture into the flour mixture. Fold gently until just blended.

5. Fold in the carrots.

6. Ladle ½ cup of batter (or the amount recommended in the waffle iron manufacturer's directions) onto the hot waffle iron. Close the lid and cook 4 minutes, or until golden.

7. Gently open lid and remove the waffle with a fork.

8. Repeat with the remaining batter, lightly coating the iron with cooking spray each time.

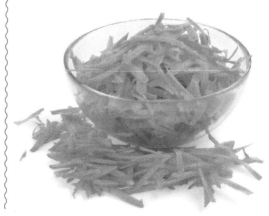

PARSNIP GRIDDLE CAKES

MAKES 6 SERVINGS

I love mashed potato pancakes but had never tried mashed parsnip griddle cakes before sampling this delicious recipe. Feel free to substitute 1 pound of carrot, turnip, rutabaga, or another root veggie for half of the parsnip.

2   *pounds parsnips, peeled*

1   *teaspoon salt*

½   *cup finely chopped onion*

¼   *cup spelt, white wheat, or gluten-free all-purpose flour, or whole-wheat pastry flour*

1   *large egg, lightly beaten*

1   *tablespoon minced parsley or other herb*

2–4 *tablespoons extra virgin olive oil for frying*

1. Place the parsnips in a large saucepan and cover with water. Add the salt.

2. Bring to a boil over medium-high heat. Reduce the heat, cover, and cook for 15–20 minutes, or until tender.

3. Drain and place the parsnips in a large bowl. Mash with a potato masher until relatively smooth.

4. Stir in the onion, flour, egg, and parsley.

5. Heat 2 tablespoons of oil in a large nonstick skillet over medium heat. Drop the batter by ¼ cupfuls into the oil. Fry in batches until golden brown on both sides, using the remaining oil as needed.

6. Drain on paper towels.

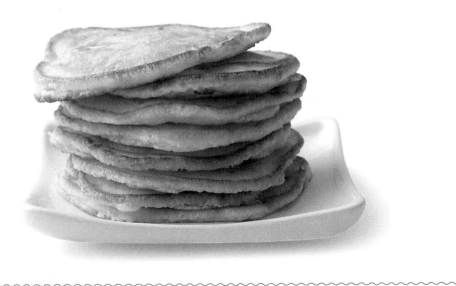

PARSNIP SALMON PANCAKES

MAKES 4 PANCAKES

This is a main-dish pancake, featuring hardworking parsnip and salmon—the superfood darling of nutritionists everywhere. Feel free to use another smoked fish if you'd like. Or leave out the fish entirely.

- 6 tablespoons coconut cream
- 1 tablespoon Dijon-style mustard
- 2 tablespoons chopped fresh parsley, or a mix of parsley and fresh dill, divided
- ¾ pound russet potatoes, peeled
- ½ pound parsnips, peeled
- 6 ounces smoked salmon, chopped
- ½ cup finely chopped onion
- 3 tablespoons chopped chives, or a mix of chives and fresh dill, divided

Salt and pepper, to taste

- 1 large egg, beaten
- 4 tablespoons extra virgin olive oil
- 12 thin slices smoked salmon (about 6 ounces)

1. Whisk together the coconut cream, mustard, and 1 tablespoon parsley in a small bowl. Set aside. This will be the garnish.

2. Coarsely grate the potatoes and parsnips into a medium bowl. Mix in the chopped salmon, onion, 2 tablespoons of chives, the remaining 1 tablespoon of parsley, salt, and pepper.

3. Stir in the egg.

4. Divide the potato mixture into four equal portions.

5. Heat 1 tablespoon of oil in a medium skillet over medium heat.

6. Add 1 portion of the potato mixture to the skillet and flatten to a 5-inch round. Cook until golden brown on the bottom, about 5 minutes. Turn the pancake over and cook until brown on the bottom and cooked through, about 5 more minutes.

7. Repeat with the remaining three portions, adding 1 tablespoon of oil to the skillet for each pancake.

8. Dress with coconut-mustard cream and the remaining 1 tablespoon of chives.

ROASTED BEET WAFFLES

MAKES ABOUT 5 SERVINGS

I grew up in a family that owned—and frequently used—a waffle iron. I still think of these waffles as the ultimate breakfast luxury. This version, in addition to being luxurious, is healthy thanks to the beets, coconut milk, and oil. Feel free to substitute parsnip, carrot, or sweet potato for some or all of the beets.

2 *large red beets*

1 *cup coconut milk*

1 *cup whole-wheat pastry or gluten-free all-purpose flour*

1½ *teaspoons baking powder*

1 *large egg*

6 *tablespoons liquid coconut oil*

Pinch of salt

1 *tablespoon coconut sugar or regular sugar*

1. Roast the beets in the oven for an hour at 400°F, covered. Let completely cool, then peel. You can save time by doing this step a day or more ahead of time. Preheat a waffle iron to 200°F.

2. In a blender, puree together the coconut milk and beets.

3. Pour the mixture into a bowl and stir in the remaining ingredients. The batter will be thick.

4. Ladle ½ cup of batter (or the amount recommended in the waffle iron manufacturer's directions) onto the hot waffle iron and press down the lid.

5. Cook for 5–7 minutes, or until done.

TURNIP LATKES

MAKES 8 SERVINGS
(20 3-INCH LATKES)

I love the turnip's slightly sweet, slightly sharp flavor—a flavor that does so well in this unusual latke. These are especially tasty with creamed chicken or shrimp over them.

 2 *packed cups peeled, shredded turnips (about 1 pound)*

 6 *tablespoons extra virgin olive oil or avocado oil, divided*

 1 *cup coconut cream*

 1 *large egg*

 ½ *teaspoon salt*

 1 *cup spelt or gluten-free all-purpose flour*

1. Place the turnips in a medium bowl and toss with 2 tablespoons of the oil. Set aside.

2. In a large bowl, beat the coconut cream with the egg and salt.

3. Stir in the flour and mix just to combine.

4. Add the turnips and fold until evenly coated.

5. Heat a large, heavy frying pan. Coat the bottom with enough of the reserved oil to prevent sticking.

6. For each latke, spread a heaping spoonful of batter on the bottom of the frying pan to form a 3-inch cake. Fry, turning once, until both sides are a deep brown, about 5 minutes per side.

If Wishes Were Horses

If wishes were horses, beggars would ride.
If turnips were watches, I would wear one by my side.
And if "ifs" and "ands"
Were pots and pans,
There'd be no work for tinkers!

—MOTHER GOOSE

BREAKFAST ENTREES

CABBAGE-CARROT FRITTATA WITH ROSEMARY

MAKES 8 SERVINGS

Frittatas are crazy-easy and a great dish to make for a crowd. If you've never made one before, give this one a try. You can use the vegetables listed below, or simply try whatever cooked veggies you have on hand.

Coconut oil to oil the pan

½ cup to 1 cup cooked (or leftover roasted) chopped beets, carrots, rutabaga, turnip, sunchoke, or parsnip

½–1 cup cubed cooked potatoes or sweet potatoes

Salt and pepper, to taste

8 eggs

2 teaspoons rosemary, chives, parsley, or other fresh herb

1. Preheat the oven to 350°F.

2. Oil an 11×7-inch baking pan, or something of a similar size.

3. Scatter the chopped cooked vegetables and potatoes in the baking pan. Sprinkle with salt and pepper.

4. In a large bowl, whisk the eggs and herbs to blend. Season with salt and pepper.

5. Pour the egg mixture over the vegetables.

6. Place the pan in the oven and cook for 15 minutes, or until the eggs are firm.

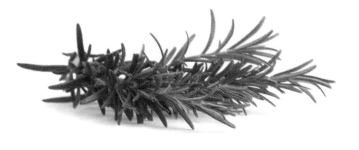

CELERIAC HASH

MAKES 4 SERVINGS

Celeriac is not a commonly used veggie in the United States, Canada, or Australia. It is frequently used in Europe, where it is grated, roasted, pureed, boiled, and much more. Here, it is enjoyed in hash. If you don't eat bacon (which goes so well with celeriac), leave it out, or substitute a cup of beans.

3 tablespoons extra virgin olive oil

1 large celeriac, peeled, cut into ¾-inch cubes

1 pound sweet potatoes, peeled, cut into ¾-inch cubes

1 cup chicken broth

1 teaspoon dried thyme

¼ teaspoon cayenne pepper

1 red onion, sliced

1 garlic clove, minced

Salt and pepper, to taste

10 slices bacon, cooked and roughly chopped

1. Warm the oil in a large pan over high heat. Add the celeriac and sweet potato and cook for 2 minutes to brown the vegetables. They will still be firm.

2. Add the chicken broth, thyme, and cayenne and cook until vegetables are just beginning to soften and liquid has evaporated, 15–20 minutes. (Add another teaspoon or two of oil if the vegetables are beginning to stick.)

3. Add the onion, garlic, and salt and pepper. Toss the ingredients often to loosen any browned bits. Cook until the vegetables are tender, about 25–30 minutes.

4. Turn off the heat and stir in the bacon.

FIVE EASY WAYS TO ENJOY CELERIAC

1. Peel and grate a small celeriac root. Dress with your favorite vinaigrette. Voilà: An easy salad!

2. Next time you make mashed potatoes, peel a small celeriac root and boil in the same pot as the spuds. Mash and season the potatoes and celeriac as you usually would for an upscale, delicious side dish.

3. Peel and dice a small celeriac root. Use in place of one potato when roasting vegetables.

4. Peel and dice a small celeriac root. Toss into your next pot of chicken soup.

5. Peel and thinly slice a small celeriac root. Pan-fry slices in a bit of olive oil until golden for an intriguing side dish.

CLASSY HASH

MAKES 4 SERVINGS

Hash is homey, easy, and economical—just open up your fridge, dice up a bunch of leftovers, and sauté! But if you need a recipe, this upscale hash (dressed in pesto) is fun and delicious. It's nutritious, too, thanks to power-packed carrots, parsnips, and rutabagas. Don't like eggs? Leave them out!

Pesto

2   cups (packed) fresh Italian parsley leaves (from two bunches), cilantro, or a mix of your favorite fresh herbs

¼   cup extra virgin olive oil

2   tablespoons pine nuts, toasted

2   tablespoons fresh lemon juice

2   tablespoons water

1   small garlic clove, peeled

Salt and pepper, to taste

Hash

2½ cups Yukon Gold potatoes (about 1 pound), peeled and cut into ½-inch dice

2½ cups parsnips, peeled and cut into ½-inch dice

2   cups rutabagas, peeled and cut into ½-inch dice

1½ cups carrots, peeled and cut into ½-inch dice

½   cup red bell pepper, peeled and cut into ½-inch dice

½   cup chopped onions

3   tablespoons extra virgin olive oil

Salt and pepper, to taste

3   garlic cloves, minced

Garnish

4   large hard-boiled eggs (optional)

1. To make the pesto, blend all pesto ingredients in a food processor until almost smooth.

2. Chop or slice the hard-boiled eggs, if using. Set aside.

3. Preheat the oven to 400°F.

4. In a large bowl, toss the potatoes, parsnips, rutabagas, carrots, bell pepper, and onions with olive oil. Sprinkle generously with salt and pepper.

5. Roast the vegetables until tender, stirring and turning occasionally, about 45 minutes.

6. Stir in the garlic and roast 5 minutes longer.

7. Divide the hash among four plates. Drizzle pesto over each serving and dress each plate with the reserved hard-boiled eggs.

HASH: A DEFINITION

Hash is one of those funny foods that most of us have eaten, but few of us know how it originated. Consisting of shredded, diced, or chopped potatoes, root vegetables, and/or meat cooked in hot oil or fat in a frying pan, hash is a common breakfast food. Its name is derived from the French verb *hacher*, which means "to chop."

ROASTED ROOT VEGETABLES WITH HAM

MAKES 8 SERVINGS

If you have never made roasted root veggies before, I encourage you to make a pan this week. It is one of those dishes that every home cook should know how to make. Here, they are turned into a beautiful breakfast dish. Feel free to leave out the ham if you'd like.

1   *blue potatoes, scrubbed and cut into ¾-inch cubes*

1   *pound rutabaga or celeriac, peeled and cut into ¾-inch cubes*

1   *pound carrots or parsnips, peeled and cut into ¾-inch cubes*

1   *pound turnips or sunchokes, cut into ¾-inch cubes*

1   *pound radishes or jicama, peeled and cut into ¾-inch cubes*

2   *medium onions, cut into large dice*

5   *cloves of garlic, peeled*

1   *tablespoon fresh rosemary*

1   *tablespoon fresh thyme leaves*

4   *tablespoons extra virgin olive oil*

Salt and pepper, to taste

2–3 cups cubed ham or Canadian bacon

1. Preheat the oven to 425°F.

2. In a large bowl, toss all the vegetables, garlic, and herbs with the olive oil. Season with salt and pepper.

3. Place the vegetables on a single layer on several baking sheets. Roast for about 45 minutes, or until caramelized on the outside and fork-tender.

4. Toss in the ham. Roast for an additional 5 minutes.

5. Remove from the oven and allow to cool slightly before serving.

DELICIOUS WAYS TO ENJOY LEFTOVER ROASTED ROOTS

- Toss in a green salad.
- Float atop a bowl of soup. Instant croutons!
- Puree with marinara sauce for a rich pasta sauce.
- Scatter over homemade pizza just before baking.
- Tuck into a sandwich or wrap.
- Use to fill an omelet.
- Fold into a pot of quinoa or millet or other grain for a quick pilaf.
- Toss with your favorite vinaigrette for a fast root veggie salad.

SWEET POTATO AND BLACK BEAN BREAKFAST WRAPS

MAKES 4 SERVINGS

If you've read any of my other cookbooks, you know that I love black beans and sweet potatoes together. In this fun breakfast recipe, this power combo teams up to offer a nutrient-dense way to start the day. As written, the recipe is gluten-free (thanks to the collard leaf wraps), but if you have a favorite wrap you'd like to use, go ahead and spoon the filling into them.

NOTE: I usually leave out the egg or sub in an organic sausage.

- 4   collard leaves
- 3   tablespoons extra virgin olive oil, divided
- 1   medium white (or orange or purple) sweet potato, peeled and chopped into ½-inch cubes
- 1   small yellow onion, diced
- Salt and pepper, to taste
- 3   scallions, chopped
- 6   large eggs, well beaten
- ¼   cup cilantro
- 1   cup cooked black beans (I used canned)
- 4   tablespoons salsa, plus more for serving
- 1   large avocado, peeled and sliced

1. Wash the collard leaves and pat them dry.

2. Remove the stems and cut out the tough lower parts of the ribs.

3. Lay the leaves on a flat surface, such as a clean counter or cutting board. Set aside.

4. Warm 2 tablespoons of the olive oil in a skillet over medium heat. Add the sweet potato, onion, salt, and pepper and cook, stirring frequently until the veggies have softened, about 20–25 minutes. If the potatoes are not soft, you can add a tablespoon of water or broth or tomato juice to help steam them.

5. In a separate skillet, heat the remaining 1 tablespoon of olive oil over medium heat. Add the scallions and sauté until fragrant, about 2 minutes. Add the eggs and cilantro and allow them to sit and firm up for 1 minute. Use a spatula to scramble the eggs to the desired doneness.

6. Divide the scrambled eggs among the collard leaves. Add ¼ cup of black beans to each collard leaf, followed by salsa, sliced avocado, and cooked sweet potatoes. Wrap the collards like a burrito and enjoy!

SWEET POTATO HASH WITH EGGS

MAKES 4 SERVINGS

This is one of my favorite hash recipes. It is nutritious (thanks to the antioxidant-packed sweet potato), filling, easy, and economical. Plus, everyone in my family likes it. Take a look at the instructions before making this, as there are several steps (all of them easy). Feel free to toss in ½–1 cup of cooked chickpeas, white beans, or diced organic Spanish chorizo if you want additional protein.

6 *tablespoons extra virgin olive oil*

2 *large yellow onions, roughly chopped*

Salt and pepper, to taste

3 *large sweet potatoes, chopped into ½-inch cubes*

1½ *teaspoons smoked paprika*

1 *tablespoon (packed) finely minced oregano leaves*

4 *large eggs*

1. Preheat the oven to 450°F. Line a large baking sheet with foil or parchment paper.

2. Heat 2 tablespoons of the olive oil in a skillet over medium-high heat. Add the onions, salt, and pepper.

3. Lower the heat slightly and cook, stirring occasionally until caramelized (soft and medium brown), about 25 minutes. When done, remove from the heat and set aside.

4. While the onions are cooking, toss the sweet potatoes, the remaining 4 tablespoons of oil, salt and pepper to taste, paprika, and oregano in a large bowl. Stir in the onions.

5. Spread the sweet potato mixture on a prepared baking sheet and roast for 25–40 minutes, stirring every 10–15 minutes, until the sweet potatoes are soft and browned. Remove from the oven.

6. Reduce the oven temperature to 425°F. Transfer the sweet potato mixture to a 9×13-inch baking dish.

7. Make small wells in the sweet potato mixture and crack in the eggs. Sprinkle lightly with salt and pepper.

8. Put the baking dish in the oven and bake for 10–20 minutes, or until the eggs are baked to your desired doneness.

9. Adjust the seasonings and serve.

BREAKFAST SIDES

BRUNCH SALAD

I am a big fan of salad for breakfast. You get a beautiful dose of energizing chlorophyll in the greens, fiber, and a wide range of antioxidants. This one, thanks to the salmon, also provides protein. Feel free to swap in an equal amount of beans, poultry, or other protein if you desire.

2   baby beets or radishes, thinly sliced

8   thin slices red onion

6   cups mesclun

2   tablespoons fresh lemon juice

2   tablespoons olive oil

1   tablespoon chopped capers

Salt and pepper, to taste

3   ounces smoked salmon or gravlax, coarsely chopped

1. Toss the beets, onion, mesclun, lemon juice, oil, and capers in a large bowl. Season with salt and pepper.

2. Add the salmon and gently toss to combine.

3. Mound the salad onto plates and serve.

ROOTY ROLLED OAT RISOTTO

MAKES 6 SERVINGS

Risotto for breakfast? Risotto made with oats? Savory oatmeal? This recipe always brings up incredulous questions. Therefore, let me say it here: The answer to any question you may have is yes. It is not only possible, but encouraged! This breakfast dish is packed with fiber, protein, and antioxidants and it is so filling and nutritious. Give it a try! (You can even serve it for dinner if you'd like.)

Sweet Potato

2   cups diced peeled sweet potato

1   tablespoon olive oil

½   teaspoon chopped fresh sage

¼   teaspoon salt

Dash of freshly ground black pepper

Risotto

5   cups chicken or vegetable broth

1½ tablespoons olive oil, divided

¾   cup diced onion

2   garlic cloves, minced

2   cups steel-cut oats

1   cup dry white wine (or an additional cup of broth)

2   teaspoons chopped fresh sage

¼   teaspoon freshly ground black pepper

4   cups sliced cremini mushrooms (about 1 pound)

½   teaspoon salt

Coarsely ground black pepper (optional)

1. Preheat the oven to 400°F.

2. To prepare the sweet potatoes, combine them with the olive oil, sage, salt, and pepper on a baking pan and toss well to coat. Bake for 20 minutes, or until tender and beginning to brown, stirring every 7 minutes. Set aside.

3. To prepare the risotto, bring the broth to a simmer in a medium saucepan, but do not boil. Keep warm.

4. Heat 1 tablespoon of the olive oil in a sauté pan over medium-high heat. Add the onion and garlic, and sauté 3 minutes, or until golden.

5. Add the oats and cook 3 minutes, or until the oats become fragrant and begin to brown, stirring constantly.

6. Add the wine and cook 1 minute, or until the liquid is nearly absorbed, stirring constantly.

7. Stir in 1 cup of the warm broth and cook 4 minutes, or until the liquid is nearly absorbed, stirring constantly.

8. Add the remaining broth, ½ cup at a time, stirring constantly until each portion of the broth is absorbed before adding the next (about 25 minutes).

9. Remove the risotto from the heat and stir in the sage and ¼ teaspoon pepper.

10. Using another sauté pan over medium-high heat, add the remaining ½ tablespoon of olive oil, mushrooms, and salt. Sauté 3 minutes, or until tender and beginning to brown.

11. Stir in the sweet potato and cook 1 minute, or until thoroughly heated.

12. Spoon about ⅔ cup of risotto into each of 6 bowls; top each serving with ½ cup mushroom mixture and black pepper.

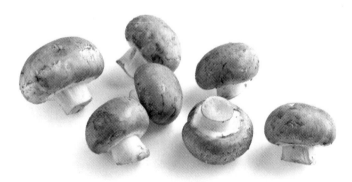

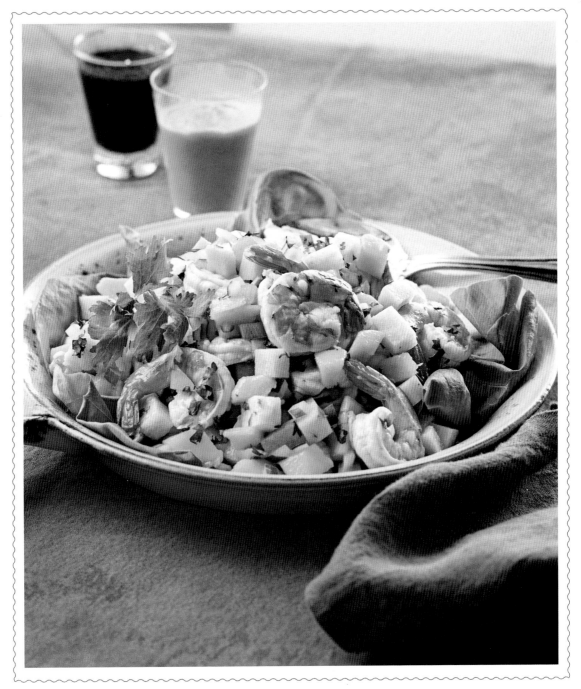

Tropical Shrimp Salad with Roots, page 126

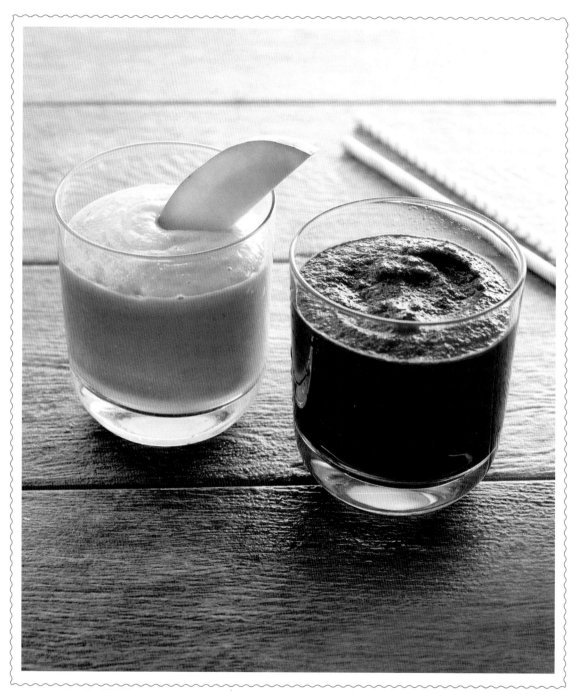

Carrot–Mango Lassi (p.45) and Red Smoothie (p.46)

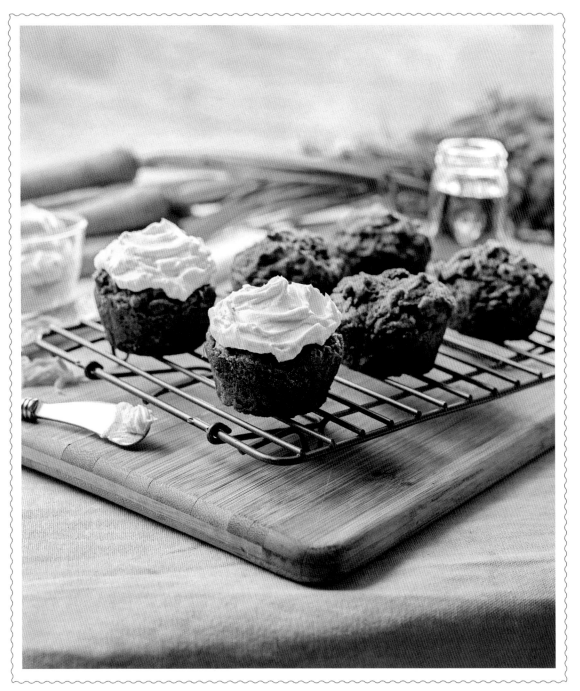

Carrot Cake Muffins, page 52

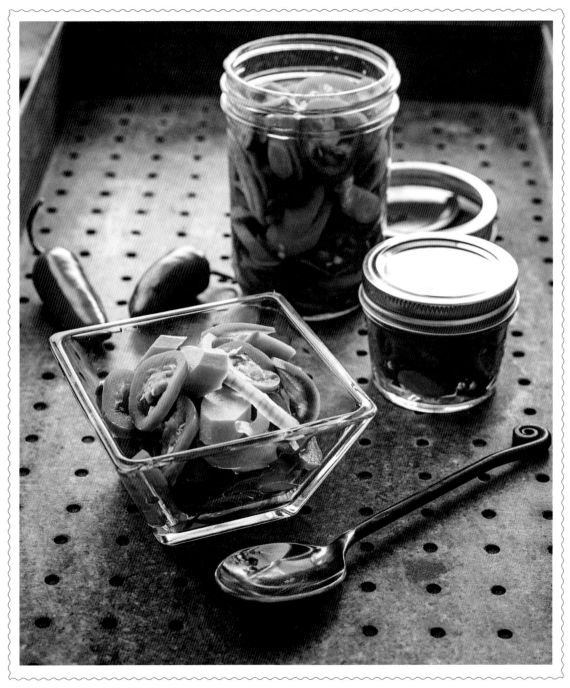

Mexican Pickled Carrots and Jalapeños, page 107

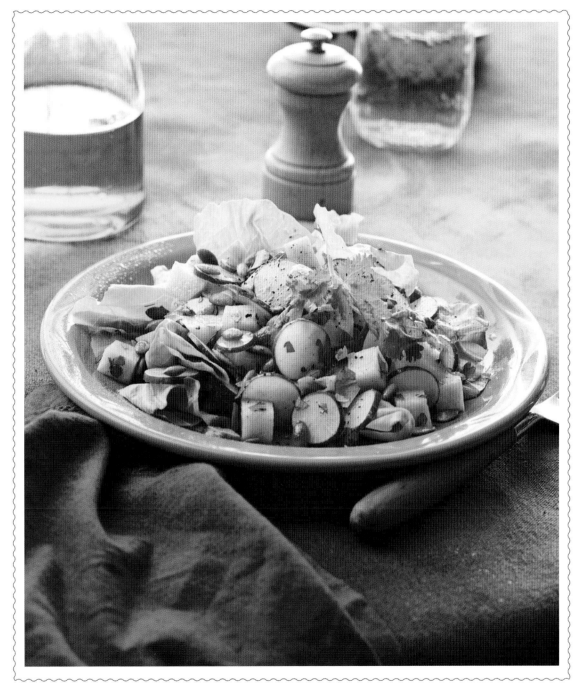

Jicama, Radish, and Pepita Salad, page 90

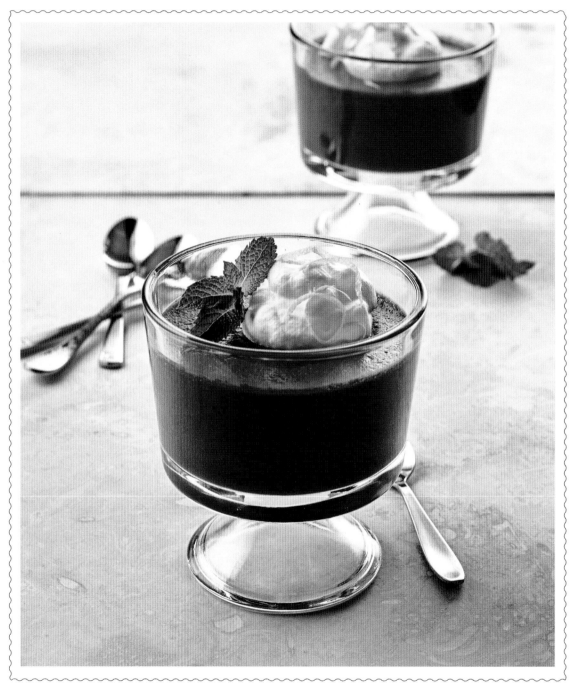

Beet Panna Cotta, page 154

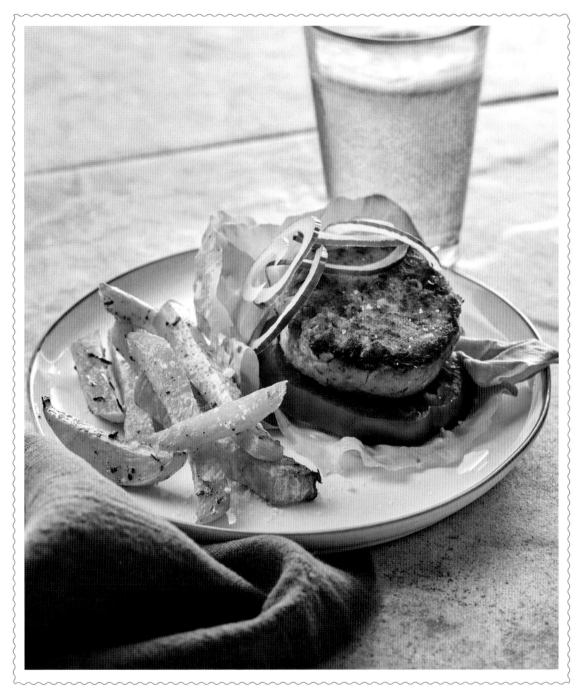

Sweet Potato Protein Burgers with Rutabaga Fries, pages 82 and 80

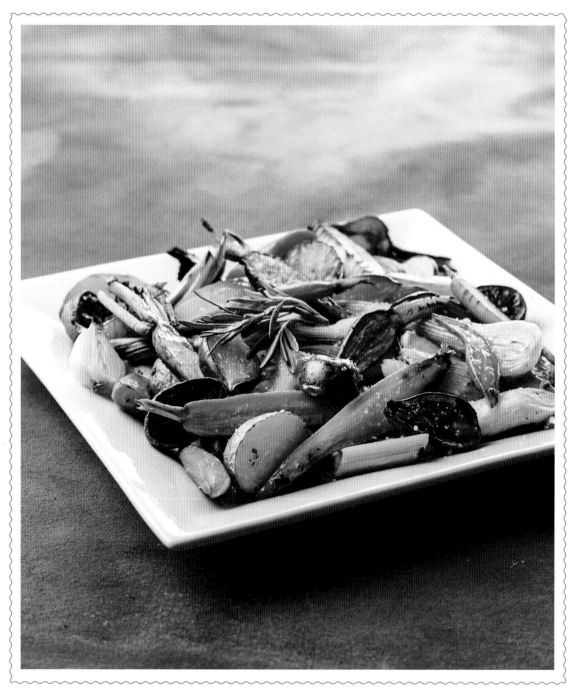

Roasted Root Vegetables, page 136

WHAT'S ON THE SIDE?

Breakfast side dishes can be anything you'd like them to be. From a refreshing green salad to a piece of fruit, side dishes can round out the morning meal with whatever sounds yummy to you. But if you need some suggestions, I am always happy to provide a few. Consider these root-themed sides:

- Grated carrot salad. To make, simply grate a carrot or two and toss with a drizzle of your favorite vinaigrette. Chopped scallions, nuts, or herbs are optional garnishes.

- Shredded roots cooked in a bit of oil and seasoned with salt and your favorite herb or spice. For a sweet side, cook in butter or coconut oil and dress with a bit of sweetener and cinnamon.

- A plate of carrot sticks. Seriously. I serve carrot sticks as a breakfast side in my household.

- Celeriac salad made with shredded celeriac and just enough unflavored yogurt (regular, Greek) or coconut cream to moisten. Season with salt, pepper, and, if you have it, parsley.

- Roasted sunchokes. These are great with bacon or sausage and eggs. See the recipe on page 136.

- Mashed rutabaga seasoned any way you'd like, packed into oiled muffin tins, and baked for 15 minutes at 350°F. These make a nice side for savory breakfasts and are cute on a brunch table.

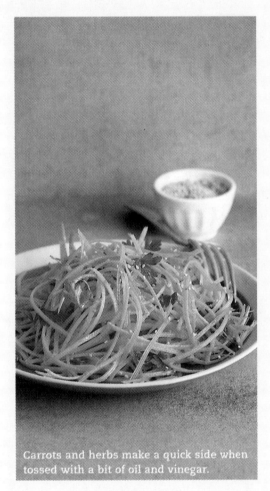

Carrots and herbs make a quick side when tossed with a bit of oil and vinegar.

WARM ROOT SALAD

MAKES 4 SERVINGS

I adore warm salads. They're so elegant and so easy, and such a fun way to serve veggies! If you've never made a warm salad, do give this one a try. Leftovers are great when added to a green salad.

1   *small red onion, cut into ½-inch wedges*

1   *small sweet potato, cut into 1-inch pieces*

1   *carrot, peeled and cut into ¾-inch rounds*

1   *parsnip, peeled and cut into ¾-inch pieces*

1   *small celeriac, peeled and cut into ¾-inch pieces*

1   *small beet, peeled and cut into ¾-inch pieces*

3   *tablespoons extra virgin olive oil, divided*

Salt and freshly ground pepper, to taste

¼   *cup pecans or another favorite nut*

1½ *teaspoons balsamic vinegar*

1½ *teaspoons fresh lemon juice*

½   *teaspoon Dijon mustard*

2   *tablespoons flat-leaf parsley*

1. Preheat the oven to 425°F.

2. In a roasting pan, toss the onion, sweet potato, carrot, parsnip, celeriac, and beet with 2 tablespoons of the olive oil.

3. Season the vegetables with salt and pepper and roast for about 45 minutes, stirring once or twice, or until tender and lightly browned in spots.

4. Meanwhile, spread the pecans in a skillet and dry-toast over medium heat until fragrant and lightly toasted, about 6 minutes.

5. Allow the pecans to cool and chop coarsely. Set aside.

6. In a large bowl, whisk together the balsamic vinegar, lemon juice, mustard, and the remaining 1 tablespoon of olive oil. Fold in the parsley.

7. Season with salt and pepper.

8. Add the vegetables and the pecans to the dressing and toss.

9. Serve the salad warm or at room temperature.

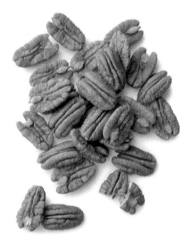

PORRIDGES, PUDDINGS, AND HOT CEREALS

AUTUMN SPICE OATMEAL

MAKES 2 SERVINGS

Oatmeal is the quintessential breakfast food for many people. It's got fiber, it's heavy and filling, and it's economical and easy-to-make, too. Here, it's dressed for autumn with sweet potato and spice.

1¾ cups water

1 cup old-fashioned oats

Dash of salt

½ cup sweet potato puree or mashed sweet potato

2–3 tablespoons maple syrup (amber or dark), coconut nectar, date paste, or other sweetener of choice

½ teaspoon ground cinnamon

Nondairy or dairy milk

3 tablespoons chopped nuts or seeds of your choice

1. Bring the water to a boil in a small saucepan. Add the oats and salt and reduce the heat to medium. Continue cooking until the oats have absorbed most of the water, about 5 minutes.

2. Stir in the sweet potato puree, sweetener, and cinnamon to combine.

3. Taste and adjust the seasonings as desired. To thin, add a splash of milk.

4. Divide the oats between two serving bowls and sprinkle with nuts or seeds.

BREAKFAST QUINOA

MAKES 2 SERVINGS

While we don't eat a ton of oatmeal in our home, we do enjoy Breakfast Quinoa frequently. Here is one of our favorite ways to enjoy this protein-packed favorite. If you happen to have a bag of millet sitting around, you can use it in the same measure for quinoa.

½ cup coconut milk (or another type of milk)

½ cup water

Salt

½ cup uncooked quinoa, rinsed and drained

⅓ cup sweet potato, carrot, or beet puree

2 tablespoons pure maple syrup, amber or dark

½ teaspoon vanilla extract

1 teaspoon pumpkin pie spice

2–4 tablespoons chopped nuts, seeds, and/or dried shaved coconut

1. Bring milk, water, and a dash of salt to a boil in a small to medium saucepan.

2. Add the quinoa, cover, reduce the heat to a simmer, and let cook 15 minutes.

3. Remove from the heat and let stand 5 minutes. Uncover and fluff with a fork, then stir in the sweet potato, maple syrup, vanilla, pumpkin pie spice, and a second small pinch of salt.

4. Taste and adjust the seasonings and sweetener.

5. Divide into two bowls and top with nuts, seeds, and/or coconut.

BREAKFAST TAPIOCA

MAKES 2 SERVINGS

Tapioca is cassava root that has been dried and ground, which is why you are reading a recipe for tapioca pudding in this cookbook. Tapioca pudding makes a lovely breakfast or brunch dish.

½ cup tapioca, soaked overnight in water

1⅓ cups coconut milk

1 teaspoon vanilla extract

1 tablespoon coconut oil, plus more as needed

2 tablespoons runny honey, coconut nectar, or other sweetener

¼ cup or more cut fruit of choice, chopped nuts, seeds, and/or dried coconut (optional)

1. Drain the soaked tapioca. Place it in a saucepan with the coconut milk, vanilla, and coconut oil. Bring to a boil, turn the heat to low, stir in the sweetener, and simmer for another 10 minutes.

2. Turn off the heat and allow the pudding to sit for 30 minutes to thicken.

3. Spoon into two serving bowls.

4. If desired, garnish with your choice of fruit, nuts, seeds, and/or dried coconut before serving.

CARROT CAKE OATMEAL

MAKES 2 SERVINGS

This oatmeal recipe features shredded or grated carrots. As my kids don't like big flakes of carrot, I make this recipe after juicing carrots, using that beautiful fine pulp that is left behind. For something different, try using pulp from yellow, white, or purple carrots. Parsnip works well here, too.

1 small carrot, peeled and shredded (about ¼ cup, packed)

1½ cups hot water

½ cup old-fashioned oats

2 tablespoons unsweetened dried coconut

2 tablespoons chopped nuts or seeds of choice, divided

½ teaspoon ground cinnamon

1 teaspoon pumpkin pie spice

Dash of salt

1 tablespoon honey or maple syrup (amber or dark) or sweetener of choice

½ teaspoon pure vanilla extract

2 tablespoons coconut milk

1. Add the carrot and water to a small saucepan and bring to a boil over medium heat. Boil, uncovered, for 3 minutes.

2. Stir in the oats, coconut, 1 tablespoon of the nuts, cinnamon, pumpkin pie spice, and salt. Cook until the oats absorb the liquid, about 1 minute.

3. Turn off the heat and stir in the honey and vanilla.

4. Transfer to two serving bowls, and top with coconut milk and the remaining 1 tablespoon of nuts or seeds.

RAINBOW OATMEAL

Want a fun way to dress up your morning porridge? Instead of cooking oats in water, substitute carrot juice or beet juice. I do this for my kids once in a while. They love the bright color, and I love the antioxidants that root veggie juice provides.

GRAIN-FREE PORRIDGE

MAKES 4 SERVINGS

I received this recipe from a Paleo friend. Outrageously protein-heavy (with not a trace of grain), it is a rich, nourishing breakfast food. It's also very delicious!

½ cup raw cashews

½ cup raw almonds

½ cup raw pecans

Salt

½ cup pureed (cooked) or shredded (raw) beet or carrot or sweet potato or parsnip

2 cups coconut milk

2 teaspoons cinnamon

1. Place the nuts in a large bowl and sprinkle a dash of salt over them. Fill the bowl with water so the nuts are covered by at least 1 inch of water. Cover and soak overnight.

2. Drain the nuts and rinse two or three times, until the water runs clear.

3. Add the drained nuts to a food processor or high-speed blender. Blend the nuts with the vegetables, coconut milk, and cinnamon until smooth.

4. Place the porridge into a pot and heat on the stove over medium heat until just warm, about 5 minutes.

5. Serve.

OATS VS. OATS

Oats come in a lot of different forms. Here's a quick rundown of the different forms this grain often takes:

OAT GROATS: Chunky and hearty, oat groats make a filling porridge and also are great cooked in broth as a savory dinner side dish. (**NOTE:** They take the better part of an hour to cook!) The word *groat* means "kernel of grain." Oat groats are oats that have been harvested and hulled. If you can't find them in mainstream supermarkets, head to a health food store.

STEEL-CUT OATS, AKA IRISH OATMEAL: This popular style of oats starts with groats that are cut into three pieces with a sharp blade. They are as hearty and delicious as groats, but take less time to cook.

SCOTTISH OATS: My kids' favorite, Scottish oats are groats that have been stone-ground (instead of cut with a blade), giving them an uneven, flaked appearance. Porridge made with Scottish oats is as hearty as its Irish relative but also has a luxurious, almost creamy, texture.

OLD-FASHIONED OATS: These are groats that have been softened with steam, rolled into flakes, then dried and packaged. These are the oats most of us grew up using to bake cookies and cooking into breakfast porridge. They are just as filling and hearty enough but lighter (and faster-cooking) than their Anglo cousins.

INSTANT OATS, AKA QUICK OATS: If you roll the oat flakes thinner than you would for old-fashioned oatmeal, you create quick, or instant, oats. The nutrition stays pretty much the same (these are all whole grains), with a slight loss of fiber, iron, and calcium. The big difference is the change in texture—instant oats are smoother, gummier (with an almost slimy quality), and much faster cooking, often needing only to be stirred with hot water to soften.

OAT FLOUR: This whole-grain flour is made by pulverizing groats. It can be used in baking and to thicken sauces.

OAT BRAN: This is the outer hull of the grain (bran) without the germ or endosperm, which is included in all the oat products above. It is not considered a whole grain.

SWEET ROOT CHIA PUDDING

MAKES 4 SERVINGS

I think I have a chia pudding in every cookbook I've ever written. The version for this cookbook is filled with sweet potato, coconut, maple, and spice. Yum! It is also packed with protein, fiber, omega-3 fatty acids, vitamins, minerals, and phytonutrients—all in one sweet dish! **NOTE:** You need to start this the day before you want to eat it. **AND ANOTHER NOTE:** You'll need to make the half cup of puree before you start. I simply toss a leftover baked or boiled or sautéed beet, sweet potato, carrot, or parsnip into a food processor and process until smooth. You'll need one medium sweet potato or beet or two medium carrots or parsnips to make a half cup of puree.

¼ cup chia seeds

1 14-ounce can full-fat coconut milk

½ cup pureed (cooked) beet, carrot, parsnip, or sweet potato

1 teaspoon pumpkin pie spice

1 teaspoon vanilla extract

2 tablespoons maple syrup (amber or dark) or other sweetener (optional)

1. In a large sealable container, stir together the chia seeds, coconut milk, root puree, pumpkin pie spice, vanilla, and maple syrup (if using). Cover and refrigerate overnight.

2. Right before serving, stir the chia seed pudding to make sure there aren't any big clumps, and then spoon into four serving dishes.

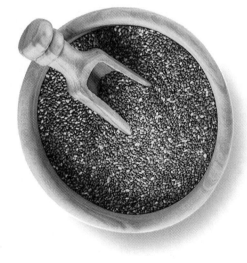

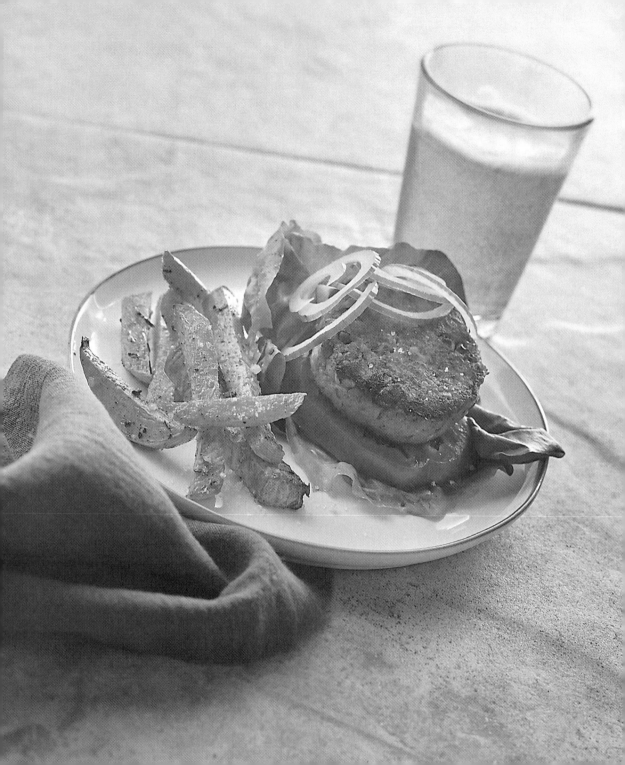

CHAPTER 4

LUNCH

Lunch is the time when your body needs the most nourishment. You've been up for a few hours and have burned through whatever calories you consumed at breakfast. It's a chance to give yourself the nutrients you need to get through the rest of your day in an energetic, calm, focused, creative way—nutrients that will boost your immune system (especially important if you happen to be around anyone who may be sneezing or coughing!), keep your heart strong, nourish your brain, ward off the threat of cancer, and prevent any sugar or carb cravings that may sneak up on you later in the day. Roots can give all this to you. And because they are so versatile, it's a cinch to include a serving or two into your midday meal. Here are some of my favorite lunch recipes to help you do just that.

BURGERS AND SUCH

BEEF-ROOT BURGERS

MAKES 6 SERVINGS

While I cannot truthfully call myself a vegan, I don't eat animal products often—and when I do, it's always in small quantities. I am always looking for ways to "veggie up" meat, which is why I love this clever idea: Augment ground beef with the grated root veggie of your choice! Having grown up in Australia, land of beets-on-burgers, my favorite is grated beets. (I use the ultra-fine pulp that's left after juicing them.) If you are trying to be stealthy, however, use turnips (and opt for just 1 cup of them). Their color and milder taste make them difficult to detect in beef.

- 1 *pound ground beef*
- 1–1½ *cups finely grated turnip, carrot, beet, or other root veggie*
- 2 *tablespoons sweet onion (such as Vidalia or Walla Walla), finely minced*
- *Salt and pepper, to taste*
- 6 *rolls or hamburger buns*
- *Condiments of your choice*

1. Put the ground beef in a bowl.

2. Add the grated root vegetable, onion, salt, and pepper and gently mix until thoroughly combined. I find clean hands are the most effective tool for this.

3. Form the meat into six patties.

4. Fry, broil, or grill as you would a regular beef-based burger.

5. Place each burger on a roll or hamburger bun and dress with your favorite burger condiments.

BEET BEAN BURGERS

MAKES 6 SERVINGS

I love veggie burgers because they are heavy on fiber, protein, vitamins, minerals, and phytonutrients. In short, they are so filled with nutrients that can protect your health and heal your spirit that you may want to enjoy them several times a week.

1   *tablespoon avocado oil or extra virgin olive oil*

1   *yellow onion, diced*

3   *cloves garlic, minced*

2   *tablespoons cider vinegar*

¼   *cup old-fashioned or other style of oats*

2   *cups cooked cannellini beans, rinsed and drained*

3   *large red beets, roasted and peeled*

1   *cup millet, cooked*

1   *large egg, or ½ tablespoon chia soaked in 1½ tablespoons water*

2   *tablespoons tomato paste*

2   *teaspoons Worcestershire sauce (optional)*

Salt and pepper, to taste

6   *hamburger buns*

Condiments of your choice

1. Heat the oil in a large skillet over medium heat. Add the onion and garlic and sauté for 10 minutes, or until the onion is translucent. Set aside.

2. Add the vinegar, oatmeal, and beans to a food processor and pulse until chunky.

3. Add the roasted beets and process until smooth.

4. Add the millet, egg, tomato paste, Worcestershire sauce, salt, and pepper, along with the reserved onions and garlic. Pulse until combined.

5. Place in the refrigerator for 2–3 hours to allow the flavors to blend and the grains to absorb the liquid.

6. Form into six patties and cook on a skillet or in a frying pan over medium heat for 3–4 minutes per side, or until the burgers are slightly golden and aromatic.

7. Serve on hamburger buns with your favorite condiments.

CARROT FALAFEL BALLS

MAKES 2–3 SERVINGS

I am frugal by nature. I have no idea why, but I am. That is why it is important to me to use the carrot pulp that is left after I juice carrots. Hence this recipe. You can also use grated carrots. Or skip the carrots altogether and sub in grated beets, sweet potato, or rutabaga.

1–2 tablespoons coconut oil, avocado oil, or extra virgin olive oil, plus extra to fry the falafel

1 small onion, grated

1 medium or large carrot, grated

2 cups cooked chickpeas

1 tablespoon chopped parsley

1 tablespoon chopped cilantro

¼ teaspoon ground cumin

Salt and pepper, to taste

1 tablespoon all-purpose or gluten-free flour

2–3 pita pockets or hamburger rolls (optional)

1. Heat 1 tablespoon of the oil in a large sauté pan over medium heat. Add the onion and carrot and sauté until the vegetables are soft, about 4 minutes. Turn off the heat and allow the vegetables to cool.

2. Add the chickpeas, parsley, cilantro, cumin, salt, and pepper to the bowl of a food processor. Pulse a few times until chunky.

3. Add the sautéed vegetables to the chickpea mixture and pulse just to blend. (You want the mixture to be chunky.)

4. Add the flour and pulse to blend.

5. Test the mixture with your fingers to see if it will hold a shape. If it does not, pulse in another tablespoon of oil.

6. Remove the mixture from the food processor and form into 12 balls about the size of golf balls. You can cover these and refrigerate them up to 24 hours if you'd like. I find that they hold their shape better if they've been refrigerated for a few hours, but you can cook them immediately.

7. Add a thin layer of oil to a frying pan and heat over medium-high heat. Add some or all of the falafel balls, depending on the size of your pan.

8. Fry the balls on one side until golden, then roll onto the other side and cook until golden. Alternatively, the falafel balls can be baked in a 375°F oven for 20 minutes, turning once partway through.

9. Drain on paper towels and enjoy as-is or tucked into a pita or hamburger roll.

MY FAVORITE FRY RECIPES

Burgers and fries—they are the perfect lunch partners, made even better when they feature nutrient-heavy root veggies. Here are two of my favorite fry recipes. They're amazing with any of the burgers or sandwiches in this section, but are also healthy enough to enjoy as a solo snack.

RUTABAGA FRIES

MAKES 2 SERVINGS

1 *small rutabaga, skin removed*

1–2 *tablespoons avocado or extra virgin olive oil*

$^1/_4$–$^1/_2$ *teaspoon salt*

$^1/_4$–$^1/_2$ *teaspoon cayenne powder*

$^1/_2$ *teaspoon garlic powder*

$^1/_4$ *teaspoon dried oregano*

$^1/_4$ *teaspoon black pepper*

1. Slice the rutabaga in half, and then cut into fries. Place them in a large bowl.

2. Preheat the oven to 450°F. Line a baking sheet with parchment paper.

3. Drizzle 1 tablespoon of the oil over the rutabaga slices and toss (your clean hands will work best) until the fries are evenly coated. If you need more oil, add a small amount.

4. Add the salt, cayenne, garlic powder, oregano, and black pepper and toss again. Transfer to a baking sheet and spread out so no fries overlap. This is important. If the fries are put too close together, they will steam instead of crisp.

5. Place in the oven and bake for 15 minutes. Remove from the oven and flip the fries. Continue baking for another 10–15 minutes, or until desired doneness is reached.

6. Remove from the oven and serve immediately.

PARSNIP FRIES

MAKES 2–3 SERVING

3   *large parsnips, ends removed, peeled, and cut into fries*

1–2 *tablespoons avocado or extra virgin olive oil*

½   *teaspoon smoked paprika*

¼   *teaspoon salt*

1. Place the parsnips in a large bowl.

2. Preheat the oven to 450°F. Line a baking sheet with parchment paper.

3. Drizzle 1 tablespoon of the oil over the parsnip slices and toss (your clean hands will work best) until the fries are evenly coated. If you need more oil, add a small amount and keep adding until you feel you have enough.

4. Add the paprika and salt and toss again. Transfer to a baking sheet and spread out so no fries overlap. This is important. If the fries are put too close together, they will steam instead of crisp.

5. Place in the oven and bake for 15 minutes. Remove from the oven and flip the fries. Continue baking for another 10–15 minutes, or until desired doneness is reached.

6. Remove from the oven and serve immediately.

SWEET POTATO PROTEIN BURGERS

MAKES 4 SERVINGS

These beautiful burgers are super high in protein thanks to the quinoa, nuts, seeds, and chickpeas. They are also high in vitamin A, alpha- and beta-carotenes, and phytonutrients (thanks, sweet potatoes!). While I love these on burger buns, I'll often crumble a patty into a chopped salad for a fast, delicious nutrition boost.

- 1 cup cooked sweet potato, no skin
- 1 cup cooked chickpeas
- ½ tablespoon finely minced fresh ginger
- 1 garlic clove, minced
- 2 scallions, chopped
- ½ minced jalapeño (optional)
- 1 tablespoon fresh cilantro, parsley, dill, chives, or a combination of these, chopped

Salt and pepper, to taste

- 1 teaspoon cumin
- 1 tablespoon lemon juice
- ½ cup cooked quinoa (white or red)
- 3 tablespoons quinoa, millet, teff, or almond flour
- 1 cup unsalted sunflower seeds
- 2 tablespoons avocado or coconut oil, for frying

1. In the bowl of a food processor add the sweet potato, chickpeas, ginger, garlic, scallions, jalapeño (if using), herbs, salt, pepper, cumin, and lemon juice. Pulse until chunky and somewhat blended.

2. Transfer the mixture to a bowl, then sprinkle in the cooked quinoa and the flour. Gently fold until combined.

3. Adjust the seasonings and fold in the sunflower seeds.

4. Form the mixture into four patties and place, covered, in the refrigerator for 1 hour or more.

5. To cook, add 1 tablespoon of oil to a frying pan and heat over medium heat.

6. Add the patties and cook for about 5 minutes, until golden. Be careful to keep the heat low. If the sweet potatoes look as if they are sticking, lower the heat.

7. Turn the burgers and cook on the other side for about 5 minutes, until golden.

8. Enjoy any way you'd enjoy traditional beef burgers.

SANDWICHES AND WRAPS

COLLARD ROOT WRAP

MAKES 1 SERVING

If you frequent raw food restaurants, I bet you've come across a collard wrap sandwich. If you have no idea what I'm talking about, I am indeed suggesting you use a collard leaf as a sandwich wrap! Just a warning: Dealing with the collard leaf can be a bit fiddly. There is definitely a learning curve on this, but you'll be a pro in no time! **NOTE:** These are on the small side. If you have a big appetite, be sure to pair them with soup or a salad, or make a second wrap.

1   medium-large collard leaf

1½ tablespoons hummus or bean-based spread (see page 120 for a wonderful recipe)

2   tablespoons shredded jicama or carrot or beets

¼   cup chopped chicken or fish, lentils, or beans

1. Lay the collard leaf flat on a clean surface. Using a sharp paring knife, shave down the center stem—called a rib or spine—that runs up the center of the leaf. Do not remove it, but just shave it to make it the same thickness as the surrounding leaf. This makes the wrap easier to roll and eat.

2. Spread the hummus on the end nearest you, leaving a 1-inch border. Top with the jicama, then the chicken.

3. Fold the two sides about ½ inch toward the center.

4. Moving to the edge nearest you, begin tightly rolling the wrap, tucking in any ingredients that escape.

5. Eat immediately or wrap snugly in a piece of foil to enjoy later.

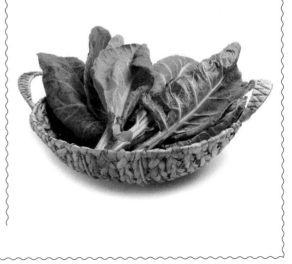

CANNELLINI VEGGIE SANDWICH

MAKES 1 SANDWICH

This sandwich practically assembles itself. It's so easy, I almost feel guilty giving you a recipe for it. But it is so deeply nutritious and so good for your heart and immune system, that I am going to get over myself and share it with you.

- ¼ cup cooked cannellini beans (or use lentils or another type of bean)
- 2 teaspoons mustard
- 1 tablespoon chopped shallot, scallion, or onion
- Salt and pepper, to taste
- 2 romaine lettuce leaves
- 2 large slices whole-grain bread, regular or gluten-free (if your bread is small, you may need to use 4 slices)
- 1 small carrot, grated
- 2 radishes, sliced thinly

1. Add the cannellini beans, mustard, and shallot to a medium bowl. Using a fork or potato masher, gently mash together the ingredients. Season with salt and pepper.

2. Place both slices of bread flat on a clean surface and lay a romaine lettuce leaf on each.

3. Add the bean mixture on top of one of the lettuce leaves on one of the pieces of bread.

4. Top with the shredded carrot and sliced radishes.

5. Cover with the remaining lettuce leaf and bread slice.

ROOT VEGGIE PITA

MAKES 1 SANDWICH

This may be one of the simplest recipes in the book, but you'll be happy to know that it's delicious as well as nutritious, thanks to the wonderful phytonutrients found in roots. If you don't have roasted root vegetables on hand, sautéed roots work, too.

- 1 large pocket-style pita
- 2 tablespoons hummus (plain or flavored; see page 120 for a great recipe)
- 2 large romaine lettuce leaves
- ⅓ cup roasted root vegetables (see page 136 for a recipe or use leftovers from last night's dinner)
- ¼ cup cooked lentils, beans of your choice, chickpeas, chicken, or fish

1. Slice the pita open just at the top. Spread the inside with hummus.

2. Add the romaine lettuce leaves.

3. Toss together the roasted root veggies with the lentils. Spoon into the pita and enjoy.

4. Because this sandwich is best eaten immediately, if you'd like to enjoy it at work, bring all the ingredients with you in a bento-style box container (don't forget cutlery!) and assemble the sandwich at your desk.

SWEET POTATO BACON (OR NOT) WRAP

MAKES 1 WRAP

This easy wrap is one I make often at home. Sweet potato, cilantro, spinach, and pepitas all work together to keep your nervous system healthy and help prevent cancer and heart disease.

⅓ cup cooked sweet potato

1 teaspoon chipotle in adobo

¼ teaspoon cumin (optional)

1 tablespoon cilantro (optional)

Salt and pepper, to taste

1 12-inch tortilla of your choice

1 tablespoon pepitas or sunflower seeds

4 nitrite-free bacon slices, cooked (regular, turkey, or vegetarian), or 3 tablespoons cooked lentils

8 baby spinach leaves

1. In a medium bowl, mash together the sweet potato, chipotle, cumin (if using), cilantro (if using), salt, and pepper. Set aside.

2. Lay the tortilla on a flat surface. Spread the sweet potato filling on the end nearest you, leaving a 1-inch border. Top with the pepitas, bacon, and spinach leaves.

3. Fold the two sides about ½ inch toward the center.

4. Moving to the edge nearest you, begin tightly rolling the wrap, tucking in any ingredients that escape.

5. Eat immediately or wrap snugly in a piece of foil to enjoy later.

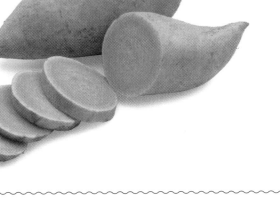

BOWLS

SUPERFOOD SALMON BOWL

MAKES 4 SERVINGS

This heart-healthy bowl features salmon, brown rice, radish, jicama, and avocado. How's that for a superfood salad?

- 2 tablespoons tamari soy sauce
- 2 teaspoons wasabi paste (from a tube)
- 2 tablespoons mirin
- 2 tablespoons rice wine vinegar
- 2–3 tablespoons sesame oil, divided
- 16 ounces wild salmon, cut in four pieces
- Salt and fresh ground pepper, to taste
- 2 cups cooked brown or red rice, warm or at room temperature
- 8 scallions, thinly sliced
- 5–6 radishes, thinly sliced
- 1 small avocado, diced
- ½ of a small jicama (or 2 small turnips), shredded
- 1 tablespoon toasted sesame seeds

1. In a small bowl, whisk together the soy sauce, wasabi paste, mirin, rice wine vinegar, and 1–2 tablespoons of the sesame oil (to taste). Set aside.

2. Rub the salmon on both sides with 1 tablespoon of the sesame oil and season with salt and pepper.

3. Place a frying pan over medium-high heat. When the pan is hot, add the salmon and sear on both sides, cooking the fish for about 4 minutes on each side. Remove from the heat and set aside.

4. Divide the rice among four bowls. Add some of the scallions, radishes, avocado, jicama, and salmon to each bowl.

5. Drizzle the dressing over each of the bowls and garnish each with an equal amount of sesame seeds.

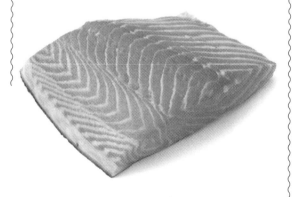

AUTUMN QUINOA BOWL

MAKES 2 SERVINGS

Every nutritionist I know adores quinoa, myself included. It's packed with protein, fiber, and minerals such as magnesium, manganese, phosphorous, folate, and iron. Plus, its light, nutty taste makes it so versatile. Perhaps this is why it's the darling of meal bowl aficionados. If you haven't tried a lunch bowl yet, this recipe is the perfect place to start.

¾ cup diced celeriac

¾ cup diced sweet potato

1 medium onion, chopped

2 cloves garlic, minced

1 teaspoon ground sage

1 teaspoon ground thyme

¾ teaspoon salt

½ teaspoon pepper

3 tablespoons extra olive oil, divided

1 tablespoon apple cider, red wine, or sherry vinegar

Pinch of sugar or other sweetener

¼ cup freshly chopped parsley, chives, dill, basil, or other herb

3 cups cooked quinoa

½ cup hazelnuts, chopped

1. Preheat the oven to 400°F.

2. In a large bowl, toss the celeriac, sweet potato, onion, garlic, sage, thyme, salt, and pepper with 1½ tablespoons of the olive oil.

3. Transfer to a baking pan and bake for 20 minutes, or until the vegetables are fork-tender.

4. Remove from the oven and let cool to warm or room temperature.

5. In a small bowl, whisk together the remaining 1½ tablespoons of olive oil, vinegar, sugar, parsley, and salt and pepper to taste.

6. Divide the quinoa into two bowls. Add the roasted vegetables and hazelnuts and drizzle with the dressing.

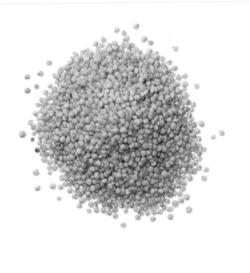

SPICY FISH TACO BOWLS

MAKES 4 SERVINGS

This yummy bowl was inspired by the fish tacos of Veracruz. Protein, omega-3 fatty acids, root veggies, other veggies—not only will this bowl keep your energy levels high, it also has plenty of great things to nourish your skin and eyes. I like to think of this as my secret beauty food.

½ tablespoon chili powder

½ tablespoon cumin

½ teaspoon cayenne pepper

½ teaspoon dried oregano

Salt and pepper, to taste

1½ tablespoons avocado or extra virgin olive oil, divided

4 4-ounce tilapia fillets (or other fish fillet of your choice)

2 cloves minced garlic

1 cup fresh or frozen corn kernels

1 red onion, diced

1 red pepper, diced

½ small jicama, diced

2 cups cooked black beans

¼ cup cilantro, roughly chopped

2 cups cooked brown rice or quinoa

4 radishes, sliced

1. In a small bowl, whisk together the chili powder, cumin, cayenne, oregano, salt, and pepper. Set aside.

2. Rub ½ tablespoon of the oil onto both sides of the fish fillets, then sprinkle the spice mixture evenly over both sides.

3. Add the remaining 1 tablespoon of oil to a sauté pan and heat over medium-high heat. Add the garlic and sauté for 1 minute, then add the fish. Sear the fish on each side, frying for 2–3 minutes before turning to cook the other side. Check the fish for doneness (it will be opaque white and will flake easily). Remove when done and set aside.

4. Add the corn, onion, red pepper, and jicama to the pan (do not add additional oil). Allow the veggies to sear without stirring. When they look browned, turn once.

5. Add the black beans and cilantro to the pan, and warm through.

6. Add ¼ cup cooked rice to the bottom of each of four bowls.

7. Divide the vegetable-bean mixture among the bowls, layer on the remaining rice, and top each bowl with the reserved fish. Garnish with radish slices.

ROOTY BUDDHA BOWL

MAKES 4 SERVINGS

Bowls are one of the trendiest things to hit midprice, healthy-food urban takeaway shops. Rice bowls, burrito bowls, quinoa bowls, sushi bowls, and here, a Buddha bowl. I've been told that it got the name Buddha after its macrobiotic-influenced ingredients (including high-nutrient burdock). I am not sure if the Buddha ate macrobiotically, but this bowl sure is good! Plus, for those of you who get a a CSA farm share, this recipe is a delicious way to use those small quantities of random veggies. Feel free to substitute other vegetables (even non-rooty veggies) for the ones I have here.

1   *burdock root, peeled and sliced into ½-inch rounds*

1   *salsify root, peeled and sliced into ½-inch rounds*

1   *large carrot, peeled and sliced into ½-inch rounds*

1   *parsnip, peeled and sliced into ½-inch rounds*

1   *large beet, peeled and sliced into ½-inch cubes*

1   *turnip, peeled and sliced into ½-inch rounds*

5   *tablespoons sesame or extra virgin olive, divided*

Salt and black pepper, to taste

4   *tablespoons tahini*

Juice of 1 lemon

1   *garlic clove, minced*

Warm water, as needed

3   *cups cooked quinoa at room temperature*

3   *cups of baby spinach, baby kale, or baby power greens*

1½ *cups cooked chickpeas, drained*

1. Preheat the oven to 450°F.

2. Place the burdock, salsify, carrot, parsnip, beet, and turnip in a large mixing bowl and toss with 2 tablespoons of the oil, salt, and pepper.

3. Place the root vegetable mixture in a single layer on a large baking sheet (or use two baking sheets to ensure the veggies are not crowded). Bake for 20 minutes, or until fork-tender.

4. In a medium bowl, whisk together the tahini, remaining 3 tablespoons of oil, lemon juice, garlic, and salt and pepper to taste. If needed, add a tablespoon or two of warm water to thin the dressing.

5. Place an equal amount of quinoa, baby spinach, chickpeas, and roasted vegetables in each bowl. Spoon dressing over each.

SALADS

JICAMA, RADISH, AND PEPITA SALAD

MAKES 4 SERVINGS

½ cup extra virgin olive oil

⅓ cup chopped fresh cilantro

1½ tablespoons white wine vinegar

1 tablespoon honey

1¼ teaspoons ground cumin

Salt and pepper, to taste

1 5-ounce package butter lettuce mix or baby spinach leaves

2 cups diced peeled jicama

1 scant cup thinly sliced radishes (about 8)

⅓ cup natural shelled pumpkin seeds (pepitas), lightly toasted

1. To make the dressing, whisk the first five ingredients in a small bowl. Season with salt and pepper.

2. Toss the lettuce, jicama, and radishes in a large bowl. Add the dressing and toss to coat.

3. Divide the salad among 4 plates. Sprinkle with pumpkin seeds and serve.

ROASTED SWEET POTATO SALAD WITH CHIPOTLE VINAIGRETTE

MAKES 4 SERVINGS

I love salads of all kinds—tossed, chopped, composed, green, raw, cooked. But I love them even more when I know they contain foods that will not only prevent illnesses, but also keep me feeling energetic and focused. This is one of those salads, thanks to the sweet potatoes, beans, and pepitas, three ingredients that provide fiber, protein, and antioxidants. Plus, the salad is super yummy and travels well. **NOTE:** It is a bit spicy. If you prefer less heat, omit the chipotle.

4 medium sweet potatoes, peeled and cut into ¾-inch cubes

1 large sweet onion (such as Vidalia), chopped

½ cup extra virgin olive oil

Salt and pepper, to taste

1 tablespoon canned chipotle chile in adobo sauce

1 small clove garlic, peeled

Juice of 2 limes

½ teaspoon oregano leaves

½ teaspoon cumin

¼ cup cilantro leaves

2 cups cooked black beans, drained (or other bean of choice)

½ cup pepitas or sunflower seeds

2–4 scallions, chopped

1. Preheat the oven to 400°F.

2. Place the sweet potatoes and onions in a large bowl and toss them with the olive oil, salt, and pepper.

3. Spread the sweet potato mixture on a baking sheet and bake until fork-tender, about 25 minutes. Set aside.

4. Combine the olive oil, salt and pepper to taste, chipotle, garlic clove, lime juice, oregano, cumin, and cilantro in a food processor or blender until liquefied.

5. Gently toss the cooked sweet potatoes, black beans, pepitas, and scallions in a bowl with the dressing until all ingredients are coated. Adjust the seasonings.

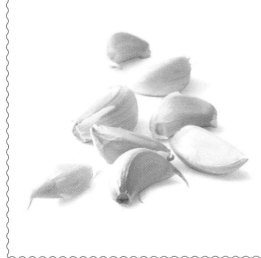

SALMON AND ROASTED ROOT VEGGIE SALAD

MAKES 4 SERVINGS

This hearty salad is perfect for an autumn lunch (or even a brunch, dinner, or barbecue). You'll see it offers some room for play. You get to pick the veggies, and no matter what you choose, you can't go wrong: All are high-antioxidant foods, helping to keep you looking young and feeling energetic, and helping to protect you from cancer, heart disease, and the common cold.

6   *cups cubed (½-inch) peeled root vegetables, such as blue potatoes, rutabagas, sweet potatoes, carrots, parsnips, and/or beets*

3   *tablespoons extra virgin olive oil, divided*

¾   *teaspoon pepper, divided*

½   *teaspoon salt, divided*

2   *tablespoons red-wine vinegar*

2   *cloves garlic, minced*

1   *teaspoon Dijon-style mustard*

8   *cups mesclun (mixed salad greens)*

12 *ounces cooked salmon (or use high-quality canned)*

¼   *cup chopped mixed herbs, such as dill, chives, and parsley*

1. Preheat the oven to 450°F.

2. Toss the root vegetables in a large bowl with 1 tablespoon oil, ½ teaspoon pepper, and ¼ teaspoon salt.

3. Spread in a single layer on a large rimmed baking sheet and roast for 25 minutes, stirring once or twice.

4. In a large bowl, whisk together the remaining 2 tablespoons of oil, vinegar, garlic, mustard, remaining ¼ teaspoon of pepper, and remaining ¼ teaspoon of salt. Reserve 2 tablespoons of the dressing in small bowl.

5. Add the salad greens to the large bowl and toss to combine. Divide among 4 salad plates.

6. When the vegetables are done, transfer them to the large bowl and gently combine with the reserved dressing, salmon, and herbs. Top the greens with the salmon and vegetable mixture.

NOTE: If taking this to work, add ¼ of the dressing to the bottom of a sealable lunch container, then add the root vegetables, salmon, and greens, in that order. Do not toss or shake. Store in the refrigerator. When ready to eat, tip the container upside down once to distribute the dressing.

SHREDDED ROOT SALAD BLUEPRINT

MAKES 2–4 SERVINGS

Rather than being a strict recipe, this is more of a blueprint for those wonderful shredded root salads (usually made with carrots) enjoyed in France. Here, I suggest one carrot, one beet, and some jicama, but it can be made with several of each or only one of these. You will be happy to know that other raw roots (radishes, turnips, and celeriac, for instance) are also lovely. A food processor with a grating attachment isn't required, but it will make this salad come together much more quickly.

1 small beet, peeled

1 small carrot, peeled

½ small jicama, peeled

½ cup cooked chickpeas

½ cup roughly chopped walnuts or pecans

2 tablespoons apple cider or red wine vinegar

2 tablespoons extra virgin olive oil

1 teaspoon Dijon or brown mustard

Salt and pepper, to taste

1. Shred each vegetable using a box grater or a food processor fitted with the grater attachment. Place the shredded vegetables in a large bowl.

2. Add the chickpeas and nuts, but do not mix them into the vegetables. Set aside.

3. In a small bowl, whisk together the vinegar, oil, mustard, salt, and pepper. Pour over the shredded vegetable mixture and toss gently to coat everything with the dressing.

4. Enjoy right away or store in a covered container in the fridge for up to 3 days.

SPINACH ROOT SALAD

MAKES 4 SERVINGS

This is a crunchy, refreshing salad that is perfect for warm weather. Feel free to add a cup or two of chopped chicken, salmon, or shrimp to the salad for a hit of protein.

½ cup extra virgin olive oil

⅓ cup mixed fresh herbs (I like cilantro, parsley, and chives) or your favorite herb

1½ tablespoons white wine or Champagne vinegar

1 tablespoon honey

1 teaspoon ground cumin

Salt and pepper, to taste

1 5-ounce package baby spinach leaves

2 cups diced peeled jicama

8 radishes, thinly sliced

1 cup pecans, coarsely chopped

1. Whisk together the oil, herbs, vinegar, honey, cumin, salt, and pepper in a small bowl.

2. In a large bowl, toss together the spinach leaves, jicama, radishes, and pecans.

3. Add the dressing right before serving, tossing gently to coat.

SOUPS, STEWS, AND CHILIS

BEET-BEAN CHILI

6 SERVINGS

This beautiful chili is a glorious deep pink, thanks to the beets. Like many vegetarian chilis, it's high in fiber and protein, but the beets add a generous amount of powerful disease-fighting antioxidants. This is great packed in a thermos for an office-day lunch, but it can also be enjoyed with tortilla chips and salsa for dinner, spooned onto nachos, or used as a burrito filling.

2 tablespoons oil

3 medium beets (or 5 small), trimmed, peeled, and chopped

1 large red onion, finely chopped

1 large red bell peppers, finely chopped

2 teaspoons ground cumin

1 teaspoon dried oregano

1 teaspoon chili powder

3 cloves fresh crushed garlic

1 28-ounce can diced tomatoes

4½ cups cooked black or pinto beans (3 15-ounce cans), drained

1 cup vegetable or chicken broth

Salt and pepper, to taste

¼ cup fresh cilantro, chopped

1. Heat the oil in a large saucepan over medium heat. Add the beets, onion, and pepper and sauté until vegetables are fork-tender, about 10 minutes.

2. Stir in the cumin, oregano, and chili powder and cook for 2 minutes, until fragrant.

3. Add the garlic and cook another 2 minutes.

4. Add the tomatoes, beans, and broth. Turn up the heat to medium-high and heat until boiling. Reduce the heat and allow the chili to simmer for 20–30 minutes.

5. Season with salt and pepper and stir in the cilantro.

NOTE: The chili tastes best when allowed to rest overnight in the fridge.

CARROT-BURDOCK BISQUE

MAKES 4 SERVINGS

I've said it before: Carrots are the workhorses of my kitchen. They are inexpensive, easy to find at any market, and store forever (I throw them in the produce drawer and forget about them until I need them). Plus, my kids like them, I can do a million things with them, and—perhaps best of all—they are loaded with fiber, vitamin A, alpha- and beta-carotene, and a large lineup of phytonutrients that help the eyes, brain, heart, immune system, skin, and more.

Pairing them with detoxifying, immune-strengthening burdock makes this one of my favorite ways to enjoy them. It's great for rounding out a salad lunch.

2 *tablespoons avocado, coconut, or extra virgin olive oil*

1 *large onion, chopped*

5 *large carrots, peeled and chopped*

2 *burdock roots, peeled and chopped*

1 *tablespoon Madras curry powder*

1 *teaspoon cumin powder*

2 *teaspoons ginger*

½ *teaspoon cinnamon*

Dash of hot sauce or a pinch of cayenne pepper

1 *14-ounce can coconut milk*

4 *cups chicken or vegetable broth*

Salt and pepper, to taste

½ *tablespoon coconut sugar or sweetener of your choice (optional)*

1 *tablespoon minced chives, cilantro, parsley, or dill (optional)*

1. Heat the oil in a large pot over medium heat. Add the onion and sauté until translucent and soft, about 5 minutes.

2. Add the carrots and burdock and sauté until they begin to soften, about 4–5 minutes.

3. Add the curry powder, cumin, ginger, cinnamon, and cayenne and sauté for 1–2 minutes.

4. Add the coconut milk and broth. Bring to a boil, then reduce the heat to a simmer, cover, and cook for 30 minutes.

5. Allow the soup to cool a bit. Then, process with an immersion blender or, working in batches, add the soup to a blender and process until smooth.

6. Return to the pot, and add salt, pepper, sweetener (if using), and herbs (if using). Heat the soup through on low, about 2–3 minutes, to help the flavors blend.

STICK IT TO YOU

Burdock seeds are hardy, barb-like burrs, which catch on clothing. In 1941, Swiss naturalist George de Mestral came in from a hike with his dog and noticed that the dog's coat was covered with burdock burrs. For whatever reason, de Mestral removed a few burrs and studied them under his microscope. Realizing that the design would make a handy clothing fastener, he got to work creating what would become Velcro—taken from the words *velours* and *crochet*.

EASY ROOT SOUP BLUEPRINT

MAKES ABOUT 4 SERVINGS

I strongly believe that everyone should know how to make soup. That is why I give all my clients and friends a copy of this soup blueprint (I also include a version of this in most of my cookbooks). Take a look and see how you can make this recipe work for you based on whatever ingredients you happen to have in your own kitchen. Enjoy yourself!

- 1 *tablespoon extra virgin olive oil or coconut oil*
- 1 *stalk celery, chopped*
- 1 *large onion, chopped*
- 2–4 *large garlic cloves, minced*
- 2 *cups chopped root vegetables*
- 6 *cups vegetable broth*
- 1 *can (about 2 cups cooked) white beans, rinsed and drained.*

Salt and pepper, to taste

Dash of curry powder, chili powder, cumin, or any other spices (optional)

1–3 teaspoons chopped fresh herb of choice (optional)

1. Heat the oil in a large pot over medium heat. Add the celery, onion, and garlic. Stir until softened, about 5 minutes.

2. Add your chosen root vegetables to the pot and stir until softened, about 5 minutes.

3. Add the vegetable broth, beans, salt and pepper, and chosen spices and/or herbs. Allow to cook for a minute or two longer, to blend.

4. Working in batches, pour the soup into a blender until the blender pitcher is no more than half full. Puree the soup until completely smooth, returning it to the pot. Continue until all soup is blended. Alternately, use an immersion blender to puree the soup in the pot.

SIMPLE CREAM OF SALSIFY SOUP

MAKES 4 SERVINGS

This is an easy recipe and a great dish to enjoy to round out a salad lunch. Salsify gives it a chowder-like taste while providing you with fiber and important heart-protecting, anticancer phytonutrients.

1   *pound salsify, trimmed and peeled*

2   *tablespoons avocado oil or extra virgin olive oil, divided*

Salt and black pepper, to taste

1   *shallot, minced*

3½ cups vegetable or chicken broth

½ teaspoon chopped fresh thyme

¼ cup coconut milk or coconut cream

1. Preheat the oven to 400°F.

2. In a medium bowl, toss the salsify with 1 tablespoon of the oil, salt, and pepper. Spread onto a baking sheet and roast until tender, about 30 minutes.

3. Add the remaining 1 tablespoon of oil and the shallot to a large pot over medium heat and sauté until the shallot is tender. Turn off the heat and set aside.

4. Chop the roasted salsify into 1-inch pieces and place into the shallot pot with the broth and thyme. Simmer over medium heat until the flavors have blended, about 15 minutes.

5. Allow the mixture to cool a bit, then process with an immersion blender or puree in a blender or food processor until completely smooth.

6. Return the mixture to the pot over low heat and whisk in the coconut milk. Serve warm or at room temperature.

SALSIFY SOUP CROUTONS

If I float croutons on soup, my kids are a thousand times more likely not only to eat the soup, but ask for seconds. One of my favorite ways to make croutons is to skip the bread and head for the salsify (you could use a different root if you'd like to): Simply peel and cube the salsify, toss in a bit of olive oil, season with salt and pepper, and roast in a 425°F oven for 15 minutes. I save these in the fridge to garnish weeknight soup dinners, but you can also use the roasted salsify warm from the roasting pan.

SWEET POTATO–PEANUT STEW

MAKES 8 SERVINGS

I make several different versions of this stew, and it's a recipe I always share with clients. It's easy, super nutritious, and high in protein. It doesn't require meat, it travels well, and even picky kids like it. It's a good recipe to have in your culinary back pocket.

- 2 *tablespoons coconut oil*
- 2 *red sweet peppers, chopped*
- 1 *large onion, chopped*
- 2 *celery stalks, chopped*
- 6 *cloves garlic, minced*
- 2 *teaspoons ginger*
- 1 *teaspoon ground allspice*
- ½ *teaspoon cinnamon*
- *Dash of hot sauce or pinch of cayenne pepper (optional)*
- 2 *pounds sweet potatoes, peeled and cubed into ¾-inch pieces*
- 4 *cups vegetable or chicken broth*
- 1 *6-ounce can tomato paste*
- 1 *14-ounce can unsweetened coconut milk*
- 1 *cup natural peanut butter*
- 2 *tablespoons chopped cilantro (optional)*

1. In a large pot, heat the oil over medium heat. Add the peppers, onions, and celery and cook until soft, about 5 minutes.

2. Add the garlic, ginger, allspice, cinnamon, and hot sauce (if using), and cook for another minute.

3. Add the sweet potatoes, broth, and tomato paste, and bring the mixture to a boil.

4. Quickly reduce the heat to low, cover, and allow to simmer for 20 minutes, or until the potatoes are fork-tender.

5. As the soup is simmering, whisk together the coconut milk and peanut butter in a small bowl. Dip into the soup pot for 1–2 tablespoons of hot liquid, and whisk that into the coconut milk and peanut butter; the warmth will help the two ingredients combine more easily.

6. Add the coconut mixture to the soup. Stir in the cilantro and heat for 2–3 minutes to allow flavors to blend.

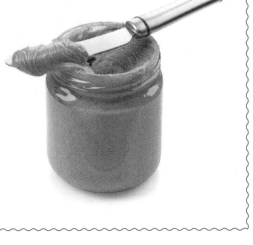

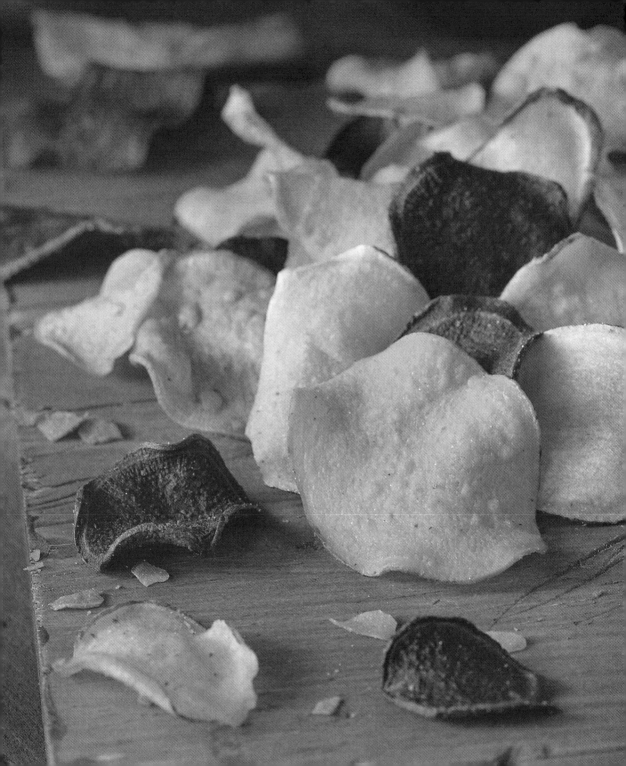

CHAPTER 5

SNACKS

S nacking is a frequent part of most people's lives. While I'm not an enthusiastic proponent of eating between meals, I understand that sometimes you just gotta crunch! That's where this chapter comes in. Short and sweet, it features a well-curated collection of root-based snack recipes. Most are easy. All are delicious and nutritious, because let's face it: If you're going to eat, why not do something that's going to improve your health and your looks (by providing you with a wide range of nutrients)? Roots can help you with both!

UNCOOKED ROOT SNACKS

GORP CARROT CHIPS

MAKES 1 SERVING

This easy snack is a veggie-style riff on Good Old Raisins and Peanuts—aka GORP, one of the few snacks we had in my house growing up. You can use jicama or turnip in this recipe, as well.

- *1 large carrot, peeled*
- *1 tablespoon nut butter (peanut, almond, cashew, sunflower, etc.)*
- *1 tablespoon dried unsweetened cranberries, goji berries, or raisins*

1. Slice carrots into ¼-inch coins.

2. Spread each carrot coin with a thin layer of peanut butter and arrange on a plate.

3. Top each carrot coin with a few dried cranberries.

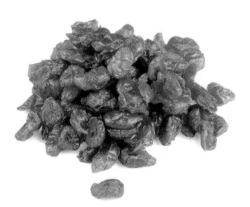

OPPOSITE: **Baked Root Chips (pages 102–103)**

MEXICALI JICAMA STICKS

MAKES 2 SERVINGS

This yummy—and healthy—treat is popular in Mexico. It is light and refreshing, and satisfies that primal need to crunch. Though not traditional, you can try this with turnip, as well.

1½ tablespoons fresh lime juice

¼ teaspoon salt

⅛ teaspoon chili powder

½ tablespoon chopped cilantro

3 cups peeled jicama cut into 3×¼×¼-inch sticks

1. Whisk together the lime juice, salt, chili powder, and cilantro in a medium bowl.

2. Add the jicama sticks and toss to thoroughly coat. Enjoy immediately.

RADISH SNACK

2 SERVINGS

This wins for the simplest recipe in the book, and it is a great way to partake in the cancer-preventative benefits of this lovely little veggie. Radishes dipped in good olive oil and salt are a popular snack in Italy. In France, butter is used.

10 radishes, trimmed or with leaves on

2 tablespoons extra virgin olive oil

2 tablespoons coarse salt

1. Place the radishes on a serving platter.

2. Place the olive oil in a small ramekin and set on the serving platter next to the radishes.

3. Place the salt in a small ramekin and set on the serving platter.

4. To eat, dip a radish in the oil and then the salt.

FIVE SNACK IDEAS FOR GRATED ROOTS

I love shredding root vegetables with my humble box grater. The roots can be used in a number of ways, including:

1. Mix ¼ to ½ cup grated carrots, beets, or other root into a tub of hummus for a quick way to create a nutrient-dense superfood spread.

2. Create a better bagel topper by stirring ¼ cup grated radish or turnip into cream cheese, spreading some on a bagel, and topping with smoked salmon.

3. I make jarred salsa healthier by stirring in ½ cup shredded jicama.

4. Shredded raw sweet potatoes are yummy stirred into a cup of vanilla yogurt.

5. Soup gets a quick upgrade when garnished with a mound of shredded veggies.

ROOTY PINWHEELS

MAKES 2 SERVINGS

Pinwheels are easy-to-make snacks that come together quickly with things you probably already have in your kitchen. They are so much healthier than chips and cookies. Use this as a blueprint, and feel free to use other spreads and veggies.

- 1 *12-inch tortilla of your choice*
- 2 *tablespoons hummus, bean dip, or your favorite nut butter*
- ¼ *cup shredded root veggies (beets, carrots, jicama, turnip, and celeriac are all good to try)*
- 2 *tablespoons chopped nuts or seeds, or cooked poultry, fish or meat (optional)*
- 2 *tablespoons unsweetened cranberries, goji berries, or raisins (optional)*
- 8–10 *baby spinach or kale leaves, or a couple lettuce leaves (optional)*

1. Lay the tortilla flat on a clean surface and spread with hummus, covering all but a ½-inch border around the circle.

2. Arrange the shredded root veggies directly over the hummus.

3. Add any additional optional ingredients you like in a horizontal line at the bottom third of the tortilla.

4. Starting with the end nearest you, roll tightly, tucking in any escaping ingredients.

5. Give the roll a squeeze to make sure everything is tightly in place, and place it, seam side down, on a cutting board.

6. Starting at one of the ends, slice off 1½-inch to 2-inch slices—pinwheels—and arrange them on a plate. This is a lot like cutting cookie slices from a log of premade cookie dough.

7. Enjoy immediately.

TURNIP SNACK

MAKES 2 SERVINGS

I love using raw veggies as the base for fun canapés. This recipe uses turnip slices. Opt for turnips that are young enough to be mild-tasting, but large enough to give you some surface area to work with. You can try this with other root veggies, too; jicama works particularly well.

4   *medium-small turnips, trimmed and peeled*

¾   *cup hummus, nut butter, or your favorite dip or spread*

3   *ounces smoked salmon or gravlax, leftover seafood or poultry, or ¼ cup cooked beans (optional)*

1. Slice the turnips into ¼-inch rounds and arrange on a serving plate.

2. Spread each slice with a small amount of hummus.

3. Top each with a small bit of smoked salmon or a bit of seafood, poultry, or a few cooked beans (if using).

COOKED ROOT SNACKS

BAKED ROOT CHIPS

MAKES 4 SERVINGS

Root chips—basically potato chips made with other root veggies—are delicious and nutritious and a surefire way to get even the pickiest eaters to eat their veggies. They are also super fun to make. Traditionally they are fried in batches, a time-consuming project. But this version is baked, which is so much easier to manage—just put the slices on a tray, pop them in the oven, and come back when they're done. You will need a mandoline or handheld veggie slicer for this recipe; using just a sharp knife will not get the slices thin enough. And yes, of course you may use different veggies from the ones I have listed. Feel free to sneak in a bit of chili powder, thyme, or other spice with the salt for flavored chips.

2   *large parsnips, peeled, skinny ends discarded, and fat ends halved lengthwise*

1   *sweet potato, peeled and halved crosswise*

2   *purple or red-flesh potatoes, peeled and halved crosswise*

1   *celeriac, peeled and halved crosswise*

2   *purple or golden beets, peeled and halved*

1–2 tablespoons avocado oil, coconut oil, or extra virgin olive oil

Sea salt, to taste

1. Preheat the oven to 375°F.

2. Prepare three baking sheets with parchment paper.

3. Using a mandoline or handheld slicer, slice the vegetables 1/16 inch thick.

4. Place the veggie slices in a large bowl and drizzle on 1 tablespoon of the oil. Toss the slices to coat. The slices should be just barely glistening with oil (you don't want them dry, nor do you want to over-oil them). If it looks like you need more oil, drizzle in another ½ tablespoon of oil and toss again. Repeat if necessary.

5. Working in batches, place the vegetable slices in a single layer on the baking sheets. Bake until crisp, about 20 minutes. Sprinkle the chips with sea salt immediately upon removing the baking sheets from the oven. Let cool on the baking sheets for 5 minutes.

COCKTAIL POTATOES

MAKES 4 SERVINGS

These are fun little potatoes eaten with sticks. My kids feel so grown-up eating these, and I feel good that they are eating a whole-food snack that is easy and economical to make.

3 pounds small purple potatoes (or use gold or red varieties)

4–6 garlic cloves, minced

¼ cup extra virgin olive oil

1 teaspoon salt

1 teaspoon freshly ground black pepper

1 teaspoon thyme, rosemary, dried parsley, or another herb (optional)

1. Preheat the oven to 400°F.

2. Cut the potatoes in half or quarters.

3. Place the potatoes and garlic in a large bowl. Drizzle the oil over the potatoes and garlic and sprinkle on the salt, pepper, and herbs (if using). Toss well to coat.

4. Transfer the potatoes to two roasting pans or baking sheets, spreading them out so they are in a single layer and not touching.

5. Bake for 20 minutes. Flip the potatoes and continue baking for 25 more minutes.

6. Remove from the heat and allow to cool slightly.

7. Spear each potato with a sturdy toothpick or cocktail pick and place on a serving platter. These are great alone, but they are also tasty served with small ramekins of ketchup, hummus, or other dips.

HEARTY CARROT JUICE PULP CRACKERS

MAKES 4 SERVINGS
(ABOUT 2 DOZEN CRACKERS)

I juice a lot of root veggies and am always looking for ways to use the dry, fluffy pulp that is left behind. This hearty cracker was developed specifically for the fine pulp of a masticating juicer.

2   *cups beet, celeriac, sweet potato, turnip, parsnip, or carrot pulp*

¼   *cup ground flax seeds*

1   *tablespoon chia seeds*

1   *tablespoon hemp seeds*

¼   *cup teff, millet, or quinoa flour*

½   *teaspoon salt*

½   *teaspoon black pepper*

Water, as needed

1. In the bowl of a food processor, pulse together the vegetable pulp, flax seeds, chia seeds, hemp seeds, flour, salt, and pepper. Pulse only until blended. The mixture should remain chunky.

2. Let sit for 15 minutes so the ingredients absorb the moisture.

3. Add water, 1 tablespoon at a time, pulsing once after each addition. Stop as soon as the dough starts to clump together.

4. Remove some of the dough and see if you can form a ball. If the dough is still a bit crumbly, pulse in another tablespoon or two of water.

5. Once a dough has formed, remove it from the processor and flatten it into a disk. Wrap it in waxed paper and allow it to rest in the fridge for 1–2 hours.

6. Heat the oven to 350°F.

7. Tear off a piece of parchment paper the size of a baking pan and place on a clean surface. Place the dough on the parchment paper and roll dough into a rectangle, about ⅛ inch thick.

8. Using a sharp knife or a pizza cutter, cut the dough into 2-inch squares.

9. Pick up the parchment paper with the cut cracker dough on it and place it on a baking sheet.

10. Bake for 40 minutes, until the crackers are firm but give slightly when pressed with your finger. Don't overbake; the crackers will harden up further as they cool.

11. Remove from the oven and run a thin spatula between the crackers and the parchment paper to loosen the crackers.

12. Transfer to a wire rack and allow to cool completely before separating into individual crackers.

VEGGIE THIN CRACKERS

MAKES ABOUT 4 SERVINGS
(24 CRACKERS)

This is another cracker made with root veggie juicer pulp. These have a light, delicate, more traditional cracker texture.

1   cup root veggie pulp

1   cup arrowroot starch

¼   cup coconut oil

½   teaspoon salt

¼   teaspoon black pepper

½   teaspoon garlic powder

½   teaspoon onion powder

½   teaspoon baking soda

Water, as needed

1. In the bowl of a food processor, pulse together the vegetable pulp, arrowroot starch, coconut oil, salt, pepper, garlic powder, onion powder, and baking soda. Pulse only until mixture is blended. It should look chunky.

2. Add water, 1 tablespoon at a time, pulsing once after each addition. Stop as soon as the dough starts to clump together.

3. Remove some of the dough and see if you can form a ball. If the dough is still a bit crumbly, pulse in another tablespoon or two of water.

4. Once a dough has formed, remove it from the processor and flatten it into a disk. Wrap it in waxed paper and allow it to rest in the fridge for 1–2 hours.

5. Heat the oven to 350°F.

6. Tear off a piece of parchment paper the size of a baking pan and place it on a clean surface. Place the dough on the parchment paper and roll it into a rectangle, about ⅛ inch thick.

7. Using a sharp knife or a pizza cutter, cut the dough into 2-inch squares.

8. Pick up the parchment paper with the cut cracker dough on it, and place it on a baking sheet.

9. Bake for 40 minutes, until the crackers are firm but give slightly when pressed with your finger. Don't overbake; the crackers will harden up further as they cool.

10. Remove from the oven and run a thin spatula between the crackers and the parchment paper to loosen crackers.

11. Transfer to a wire rack and allow to cool completely before separating into individual crackers.

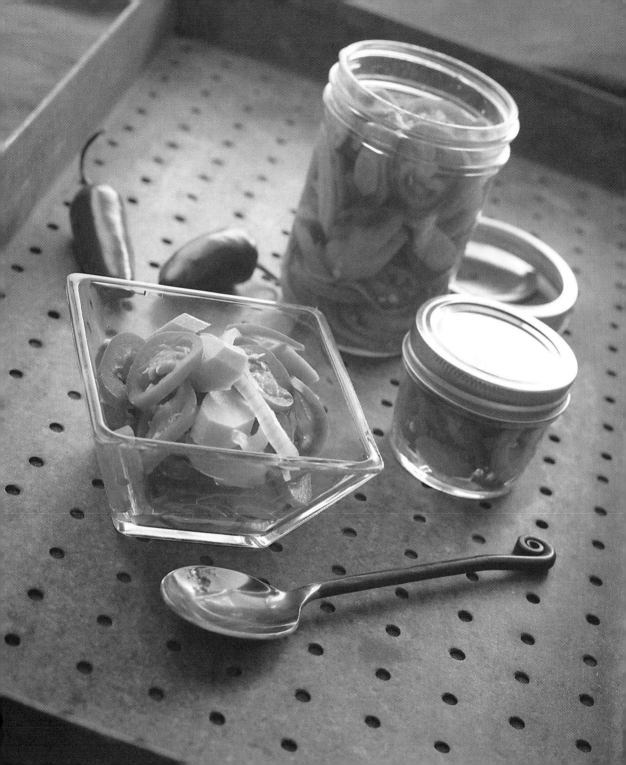

CHAPTER 6

CONDIMENTS

Root vegetables make outstanding condiments. If this sounds strange to you, think about the condiments you may have grown up with: relishes, chutneys, salsas, pickles, ketchup, and mustard—all of these are made tastier and more nutritious with sweet, earthy roots. Depending on the country you were raised in, you may already be familiar with root condiments. As a girl in Australia, I enjoyed spiced beet slices on burgers and sandwiches. Many of my friends with Mexican parents grew up eating briny carrots and jalapeños alongside grilled meats. And pickled turnips are favorite condiments in Lebanon and Turkey. Take a look at these easy, deeply nourishing recipes. I promise you'll find a few delicious favorites.

PICKLES

MEXICAN PICKLED CARROTS AND JALAPEÑOS

MAKES 2 CUPS

This is one of my favorite pickles. It is popular in Mexican homes and is fantastic alongside grilled and roasted foods.

- *1½ cups white vinegar*
- *¼ cup raw sugar or coconut sugar*
- *½ teaspoon salt*
- *10 fresh jalapeños (deseeded or not), sliced into ⅛-inch or slightly smaller rings*
- *2 cups peeled carrots, sliced into ¼-inch rounds*
- *½ red onion, sliced into ¼-inch slices*

1. Add the vinegar, sugar, and salt to a medium nonreactive saucepan over medium-high heat. Heat to a boil, then add the jalapeños, carrots, and onion.

2. Immediately turn the heat to low and allow the ingredients to steep for 1 hour.

3. Turn off the heat and allow to cool before storing in an airtight container in the refrigerator.

PARSNIP-CARROT PICKLE

MAKES ABOUT 1 QUART

Oh, wow, this is a yummy pickle! It is one of my favorite ways to enjoy parsnips (and carrots and chiles). Do give this a try. It's a bit higher in sugar than I'd like, but I haven't been able to successfully reduce it. The pickle can be used as a side or as a sandwich topper. **NOTE:** Allowing the vegetables and brine to cool separately may seem a bit fiddly, but it helps the veggies retain a bit of bite.

- 3 cups water
- ⅔ cup sugar
- ½ cup cider vinegar
- 6 whole cloves
- 6 allspice berries
- 1–2 small dried red chiles
- 1 bay leaf
- 2 teaspoons yellow mustard seed
- 1 teaspoon ground turmeric
- 1 teaspoon ground ginger
- 4 teaspoons salt
- 2 medium parsnips, peeled, cored, and cut into sticks 2 inches long and ¼ inch thick
- 2 large carrots, peeled and cut into sticks 2 inches long and ¼ inch thick
- 1 medium yellow onion, thinly sliced
- 1–2 fresh jalapeños, thinly sliced

1. Combine the water, sugar, vinegar, cloves, allspice, chiles, bay leaf, mustard seed, turmeric, ginger, and salt in a large nonreactive saucepan over medium-high heat. Bring to a boil.

2. Add the parsnips, carrots, and onion and cook for about 5 minutes.

3. Turn off the heat and add the jalapeño.

4. Remove the vegetables from the hot brine and place in a 1-quart canning jar or a sealable food container. Set aside.

5. Allow the brine to cool.

6. When both the vegetables and brine are cool, pour the brine over the vegetables, seal the jar or container, and place in the refrigerator for up to 2 weeks.

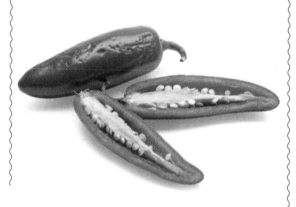

PICKLED TURNIPS

MAKES ABOUT 6 CUPS

These are always the first things I eat when I go out for Turkish food. I find their salty-sharp taste positively addictive. Traditionally, these are made pink by slipping a beet slice into the mix, but I find it's easiest to make them without the beet. If you want to give these as gifts, get three 2-cup canning jars with lids. For everyday eating, I store this pickle in a big container in the fridge.

- 1½ cups white wine vinegar or apple cider vinegar
- 1½ cups water
- 1 tablespoon salt
- 1½ tablespoons coconut or cane sugar
- 1½ pounds turnips, peeled and cut into ¼- to ½-inch sticks (about 8 cups)
- 3 whole large cloves garlic, sliced

1. Combine the vinegar, water, salt, and sugar in a large nonreactive saucepan over medium heat. Bring to a boil and stir until the salt and sugar dissolve, about 2 minutes. Remove from the heat.

2. Add the turnips and garlic to the pot and allow the ingredients to steep as the liquid cools.

3. When the mixture is cool, transfer to a sealable food storage container and store for up to 3 weeks in the refrigerator.

SUNCHOKE PICKLES

MAKES ABOUT 4 CUPS

This delicious pickle is based on an old Southern favorite. It's an easy, fun, and economical way to make something that comes across as a truly gourmet food. These are great on sandwiches and burgers, as well as eaten alongside poultry, meats, and grains.

- 2 tablespoons fresh lemon juice
- Large bowl filled with cold water
- 2 pounds sunchokes
- 1¾ cups white wine vinegar
- ⅔ cup sugar
- ¾ cup water
- ½ tablespoon whole mustard seeds
- ½ teaspoon turmeric
- ¼ teaspoon cayenne
- 1½ teaspoons salt
- ½ large sweet onion, halved lengthwise and thickly sliced

1. Stir the lemon juice into a large bowl of cold water. Set aside.

2. Peel the sunchokes and cut into ½-inch slices, immediately dropping the slices into the lemon water to prevent discoloration.

3. Combine the vinegar, sugar, ¾ cup water, mustard seeds, turmeric, cayenne, and salt and bring to a boil in a medium nonreactive saucepan over medium-high heat.

4. Stir until the sugar has dissolved, then turn off the heat and allow the brine to cool to room temperature.

5. Add water to another medium pot over medium-high heat and allow to boil. Add the sunchokes and onion to the pot and cook for 1 minute.

6. Turn off the heat and drain the vegetables in a large colander. Set aside and allow the vegetables to cool to room temperature.

7. When the vegetables have cooled, add them to a sealable container and pour the brine over the top.

8. Allow to pickle for 1 week to develop flavors, stirring occasionally to ensure all veggies get equal time in the brine.

9. Store in refrigerator for up to 1 month.

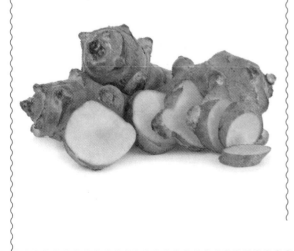

BURDOCK OR SALSIFY RELISH

MAKES 1½ CUPS

This fun recipe can be made with burdock, salsify, or scorzonera. It is savory, a teeny bit sweet, and lovely with fish of all kinds— though it's pretty darn yummy paired with cooked grains, poultry, pork, or even crackers, too.

1   *small garlic clove, minced*

½   *small shallot, finely chopped*

½   *teaspoon salt, plus additional to taste*

½   *teaspoon coconut sugar or cane sugar*

¼   *teaspoon ground black pepper*

Juice of 1 lemon

8   *ounces burdock, salsify, or scorzonera*

1   *cup dry white wine*

½   *cup water*

1   *bay leaf*

½   *teaspoon lemon zest*

1   *tablespoon extra virgin olive oil*

1–2 *tablespoons finely chopped fresh herbs of your choice, such as parsley, chives, basil, dill, or chervil*

1. Mix the garlic, shallot, ½ teaspoon salt, sugar, and black pepper in a medium bowl. Set aside.

2. Fill a separate bowl with cool water and the lemon juice. Set aside.

3. Scrub the burdock with a vegetable brush, occasionally dampening it with some cold water if needed. Upon removing the brown coating, quickly slice it into ¼-inch cubes, immediately dropping the sliced pieces into the lemon water to prevent browning.

4. In large sauté pan over medium-high heat, whisk together the wine, water, salt to taste, bay leaf, and lemon zest. Drain the sliced burdock and shake it dry. Add it to the pan.

5. Bring this mixture to a boil, then turn the heat to medium-low and cook, covered, for 30 minutes, or until the burdock is fork-tender but not mushy. The burdock should have the texture of an artichoke, soft and yielding, yet still be al dente.

6. Strain the cooked burdock mixture and allow to cool. Reserve any liquid that remains in the pan.

7. Remove the bay leaf.

8. Combine the burdock mixture with the shallot-garlic mixture.

9. Stir in any reserved liquid and the olive oil into the mixture.

10. Place in a covered container in the refrigerator and allow to rest overnight for the flavors to blend.

11. Stir in the herbs right before serving.

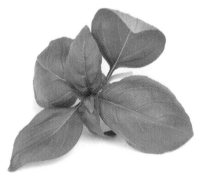

BEET CHUTNEY

MAKES 2¼ CUPS

If you like to cook, having a good chutney in your lineup will make you feel like a culinary rock star. It's easy, versatile, nutritious, and just exotic enough to make everyday meats, poultry, grains, and sandwiches feel special. This one is made with beets and cranberries. Yum!

¼ cup extra virgin olive oil

1¾ cups chopped red onion

1 2-inch-diameter beet, peeled, cut into ¼-inch cubes

½ cup water

½ cup red wine vinegar

¼ cup unsweetened cranberries

¼ cup finely chopped dates

2 teaspoons chopped peeled fresh ginger

1 teaspoon yellow mustard seeds

Salt and pepper, to taste

1. Add the olive oil, onion, and beet to a medium saucepan over medium heat. Cook until the onion is tender but not brown, about 8 minutes.

2. Add the water. Increase the heat to high and boil until the mixture is thick, about 5 minutes.

3. Add the vinegar, cranberries, dates, ginger, and mustard seeds. Reduce the heat to medium-low and simmer until the beet cubes are tender and the chutney is thick, stirring often, about 8 minutes.

4. Season to taste with salt and pepper.

5. Cool and place in an airtight jar or container and store in refrigerator for up to 10 days.

RADISH-JICAMA SALSA

MAKES ABOUT 2 CUPS

This fresh-tasting salsa is fast and so cooling—the perfect summer salsa! It is tasty with tortilla chips and in fish tacos. It's also great on grilled poultry and fish. Sometimes I add in 1–2 cups of cubed avocado.

2 cups chopped radishes

1 cup chopped jicama

½ small red onion, chopped

2 scallions, thinly sliced

1 tablespoon minced fresh jalapeño or serrano pepper

2 tablespoons freshly squeezed lemon or lime juice, or more to taste

¼ cup chopped fresh cilantro leaves

Salt and freshly ground black pepper

1. Put all the ingredients in a medium bowl and toss thoroughly to combine.

2. Taste and adjust the seasonings, adding more chile, lemon or lime, salt, and/or pepper as needed.

3. Serve immediately or keep tightly covered for up to 1 day.

DON'T TOSS YOUR CARROT TOPS

If you've ever wondered if there was something you could do besides composting carrot greens, I've got an answer for you: Yes. I juice them or mince a cup into a pot of cooking grains for a celery-parsley flavor. Another option, however, is this Italian-style fresh sauce, which is lovely with grilled and roasted foods and great on sandwiches and potatoes.

FRESH GREEN SAUCE

MAKES ABOUT 2 CUPS

Not to be confused with Mexican salsa verde, Italian salsa verde is a fresh sauce traditionally made with parsley, anchovies, capers, lemon, and flavorful herbs. Here you can use carrot tops instead of parsley, and the carrots themselves help sweeten up the accompanying mixture of starchy roasted root vegetables, a classic wintertime side dish. You'll have leftover sauce, which is fantastic with roasted fish.

5   pitted green olives (any varieties or size)

3   tablespoons capers, drained

2   whole cloves garlic, peeled

¼–½ fresh jalapeño, deseeded (optional)

1   bunch carrot tops, washed well and chopped (about 3 cups)

1   tablespoon fresh rosemary

1   tablespoon fresh chives

2   teaspoons fresh thyme

¼   teaspoon red chile flakes

2   tablespoons lemon juice

⅔   cup extra virgin olive oil

Salt and pepper, to taste

1. Add the olives, capers, garlic, and jalapeño (if using) to a food processor and pulse until finely chopped.

2. Add the carrot tops, rosemary, chives, thyme, red chile flakes, and lemon juice to the food processor and continue to process until finely chopped.

3. Gradually pour in the olive oil through the feed tube and puree until very smooth. Season with salt and pepper.

4. Store for up to 3 days in a tightly sealed container in the refrigerator.

SUPERFOOD CAPONATA

MAKES ABOUT 3½ CUPS

This recipe is a chunky dip-like dish, similar to Italian caponata. It is delicious eaten with your favorite dipper, spooned onto crostini, or draped across a dish of polenta or another grain. It's also good with poultry and fish.

- 2   small rutabagas (about 5 inches in diameter), peeled and cut into ½-inch dice
- 5   tablespoons extra virgin olive oil, divided

Salt and pepper, to taste

- 1   onion, finely diced
- 1   clove garlic, minced
- 1   shallot, minced
- ¼   cup balsamic vinegar
- ¼   cup coarsely chopped walnuts
- 1   teaspoon red pepper flakes
- 2   teaspoons coconut, raw, cane, or brown sugar

1. Preheat the oven to 400°F. Line a rimmed baking sheet with aluminum foil.

2. Toss the rutabaga with 2 tablespoons of the oil and salt and pepper to taste. Bake, turning once, for 30 minutes, or until the rutabaga is tender but still somewhat firm. Set aside.

3. In a large pan over medium heat, heat the remaining 3 tablespoons of oil. Add the onion and cook, stirring, until it is translucent, about 4 minutes, then add the garlic and shallot, stirring to mix.

4. Add the balsamic vinegar, scraping the pan to deglaze it and incorporate the addition. Add the roasted rutabaga, walnuts, red pepper flakes, and sugar.

5. Season with salt and pepper to taste.

MAKE-AHEAD VEGETABLE DIPPERS

If, like me, you're trying to limit the amount of tortilla chips, crackers, and bread you eat, you'll love this tip for using root vegetables as a healthy dipper. Take your favorite root vegetable, peel, and cut into sticks, rounds, or planks. (My favorites are parsnips, turnips, and jicama, sliced into planks.) Fill a large bowl with cold water, add 12 or more ice cubes, and submerge your prepped root vegetables. Store the entire bowl in the refrigerator for up to two days. When you're ready to dip, remove the prepped veggies from the ice water, blot dry, and use them to scoop up anything from salsa to hummus.

SPREADS AND SAUCES

BEET-DATE KETCHUP

MAKES 3 CUPS

This is a beautiful ketchup based on beets. You can use raw beets or grab leftover cooked beets if you happen to have them on hand.

1   *pound cooked red beets, diced (about 2½ cups)*

½   *cup chopped dates*

1   *cup apple cider vinegar*

¼   *cup diced onion*

½   *teaspoon salt*

¼   *teaspoon ground coriander*

¼   *teaspoon ground cloves*

Freshly ground black pepper, to taste

1. Combine the beets, dates, vinegar, and onion in a large saucepan over high heat and stir to combine. Bring to a boil.

2. Reduce the heat to medium-high and cook for 25 minutes, or until the beets and dates are tender.

3. Remove the saucepan from the heat and allow the ingredients to cool slightly.

4. In a blender or food processor, puree the beet mixture with the salt, coriander, cloves, and black pepper. Process until smooth. Adjust the seasonings as needed.

5. Keep for up to 2 weeks in a covered container or bottle in the fridge.

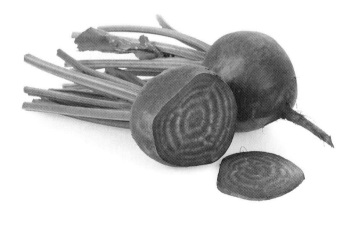

SWEET POTATO MUSTARD

MAKES ABOUT 1 CUP

Not only is this lovely mustard chock-full
of vitamin A, fiber, and phytonutrients
(thanks to the sweet potato), it's also one
of the tastiest mustards you'll ever have.
It's fantastic on hot dogs of all kinds, but
just as great on sandwiches. If you don't
have sweet potato, use the same amount
of pumpkin, beet, or carrot puree.

½ cup apple cider vinegar

⅓ cup yellow mustard seeds

1 bay leaf

1 cup water

1 tablespoon honey

⅔ cup sweet potato puree

¼ cup packed brown sugar

½ teaspoon sweet paprika

½ teaspoon kosher salt

Pinch of cinnamon

Pinch of allspice

Pinch of cayenne

1. Add the vinegar to a small saucepan over
medium-high heat. Bring to a boil.

2. Remove from the heat and add the
mustard seeds and bay leaf. Place the lid on
the pot and let sit for 1 hour.

3. Discard the bay leaf.

4. Pour the vinegar and mustard seeds into
a blender or food processor. Process until
smooth.

5. Add the water and honey and process
until smooth.

6. Add the sweet potato and process until
smooth.

7. Scrape the mixture back into the saucepan
and bring to a boil. Reduce the heat to
medium-low and simmer, stirring frequently,
for about 5 minutes.

8. Whisk in the sugar, paprika, salt,
cinnamon, allspice, and cayenne. Allow
mixture to simmer until thick, about
8–10 more minutes.

9. Remove from the heat and allow the
mixture to cool.

10. Pour into a clean bottle or covered
container and allow flavors to blend for
24 hours before using. Store in the
refrigerator for up to 1 month.

DIPS

CANNELLINI BEET DIP

MAKES ABOUT 3 CUPS

If a recipe contains cannellini beans, I am bound to love it. And if it contains beets, I will probably love it even more! Which is why I can't get enough of this cannellini beet dip. Containing protein, fiber, and huge amounts of phytonutrients, this nutritious and delicious dip is one I make often.

2   *large beets*

1   *clove garlic, minced*

2   *tablespoons extra virgin olive oil*

1   *teaspoon paprika*

1   *15-ounce can cannellini beans or navy beans, drained and rinsed*

   Salt and pepper, to taste

1. Preheat the oven to 375°F.

2. Wrap the beets in foil and place them in the oven. Bake for 45–60 minutes, or until tender.

3. Remove the beets from the oven and discard the foil. When the beets are cool, slip their outer skin off. It will come right off when you rub it.

4. Place the beets in a food processor or blender (roughly chopping or slicing them first, if you need to for fit) and process until chunky.

5. Add the garlic, olive oil, and paprika and process until blended.

6. Add the beans, salt, and pepper and process until smooth. Add about 1 tablespoon of water if needed for a smoother consistency.

7. Store in a covered container in the refrigerator for up to 5 days.

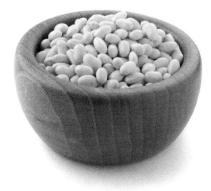

RECIPE TIP

If you have a leftover sweet potato in the fridge, go ahead and scoop out the cooked flesh and use it in the recipe as a substitute for the beets. Delicious!

CARROT SPREAD

MAKES ABOUT 1½ CUPS

This is one of my household's favorite dips. We make several different variations of it. It's healthy (beta-carotene, fiber, phytonutrients) and economical. Plus, everyone loves it. Try it with sweet potato or squash if you are out of carrots.

6 *medium carrots, thinly sliced*

½ *small garlic clove, chopped*

¼ *teaspoon ground cumin*

¼ *teaspoon finely grated peeled fresh ginger*

⅛ *teaspoon ground cinnamon*

Pinch of cayenne pepper or dash of hot sauce (optional)

1–2 *tablespoons tahini, almond butter, or cashew butter*

2 *teaspoons fresh lemon juice*

Salt and ground pepper, to taste

1. Set a steamer basket in a saucepan with 2 inches of simmering water. Add the carrots. Cover and steam until tender, about 12 minutes. Or simply boil carrots in a small amount of water and drain when done.

2. Transfer the carrots to a food processor and add the remaining ingredients. Process until smooth, about 1 minute, adding up to 2 tablespoons of water, if necessary, for a smoother consistency.

3. Adjust the seasonings as desired.

CREAMY CREAM-FREE RADISH DIP

MAKES ABOUT 1 CUP

I love creamy dips, but I loathe using mayonnaise, dairy products, or—heaven forbid—tofu to create that creamy texture. This lively dip uses cashews to give it an almost dairy-like finish. It's a great high-protein, high-fiber way to enjoy the cancer-fighting benefits of radishes. I bet you'll love this one! Try it!

6–8 *radishes, chopped*

1 *cup raw cashews, soaked in water for 30–60 minutes, then drained*

2 *cloves garlic*

1 *tablespoon lemon juice*

1 *tablespoon tahini*

Salt and pepper, to taste

1–2 *teaspoons chopped fresh parsley, chives, dill, or cilantro*

Sprinkle of cayenne pepper

1. Combine the radishes and soaked cashews in a food processor and process until crumbly.

2. Add the garlic, lemon juice, and tahini and process until smooth, adding teaspoons of water as needed to create a smooth texture.

3. Add the salt, pepper, herbs, and cayenne. Pulse until blended.

4. Store in a covered container in the refrigerator for up to 3 days.

SUPERFOOD SKORDALIA

MAKES ABOUT 3 CUPS

Skordalia is the wonderful potato-garlic (or maybe I should say "garlic-potato") dip that is beloved in Greece. Here, I've replaced the russet potatoes with highly nutritious purple potatoes, though you could also use gold or pink types.

1 pound purple potatoes, peeled

Salt, as needed

8 medium cloves garlic, minced

¾ cup whole blanched almonds

½ cup extra virgin olive oil

½ cup water

5 tablespoons freshly squeezed lemon juice

3 tablespoons white wine vinegar

Freshly ground black pepper

1. Put the potatoes in a medium saucepan and cover with cold water by about 2 inches. Season generously with salt. Bring to a boil over high heat, lower the heat to maintain a gentle simmer, and cook until very tender, about 30 minutes. Drain the potatoes and let them cool slightly.

2. Coarsely chop the potatoes, then smash with a potato masher until almost smooth.

3. In a food processor, combine the garlic, almonds, oil, and a pinch of salt, and puree into a paste. Pulse in the water, lemon juice, vinegar, black pepper, and another pinch of salt. Pulse until just combined.

4. Scrape the mixture into the potatoes and mash until incorporated. Adjust the seasonings.

5. Serve immediately. Store any leftovers in a tightly sealed container in the refrigerator for up to 2 days.

RECIPE TIP

Though skordalia is traditionally made with potatoes, I have tried turnips and parsnips. The result, though not "Greek," is very delicious. If you'd like to give this a try, substitute a pound of another root veggie for the potatoes—or use part potatoes and part another root—and continue with the recipe instructions.

SWEET POTATO HUMMUS

MAKES ABOUT 4 CUPS

My kids eat a lot of hummus, which is a good thing. It's loaded with healthy fats, protein, and fiber. But the sweet potato in this version really kicks the nutrition up a notch, thanks to the root veggie's high antioxidant content.

- 2 medium sweet potatoes
- 3 tablespoons extra virgin olive oil
- 1 15-ounce can chickpeas (about 2 cups cooked)
- 3 tablespoons tahini
- 3 cloves garlic, peeled

Juice of 1 lemon

Salt, to taste

- ½ teaspoon cayenne pepper
- ½ teaspoon smoked paprika
- ¼ teaspoon cumin

1. Preheat the oven to 400°F. Bake the sweet potatoes on the middle oven rack or in a baking dish for 45–60 minutes, until soft. Remove the sweet potatoes and set aside to cool.

2. Add the remaining ingredients to a food processor and process until smooth.

3. Remove the peels from the sweet potatoes and discard them or save them for another purpose (I toss them into the stockpot when I make broth). Add the sweet potato flesh to the food processor and process until smooth.

4. Store in a sealed container in the refrigerator for up to 5 days.

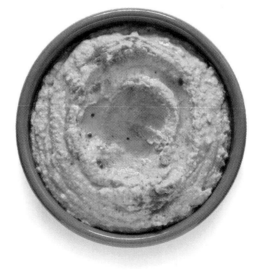

TEN USES FOR HUMMUS

Hummus is a great dip and it makes an easy, nutritious spread, but don't limit yourself! Here are some of my favorite ways to use hummus:

1. Add between ½ cup and 1 cup hummus to a 4–8 serving dish of cooked grain for a risotto-like texture.

2. Skip the red sauce! Dress gluten-free and regular pasta with ½ cup to 1 cup of your favorite hummus for an instant "cream" sauce.

3. For a juicier burger, stir in ¼ cup hummus per pound of ground meat.

4. Use as an equal replacement for mayonnaise on sandwiches and in tuna, chicken, or potato salad.

5. Thin 1 cup hummus with 1 cup broth for a quick, creamy soup.

6. Whisk together ¼ cup hummus, 1 tablespoon extra virgin olive oil, and 1 tablespoon vinegar for delicious salad dressing.

7. Slather over chicken or fish before frying or baking.

8. Make a quick sandwich by spreading bread with hummus, layering with shredded carrot or beet, and adding any other desired toppings.

9. Mix equal amounts of hummus and cooked grain, shape mixture into patties, and pan-fry for quick croquettes.

10. Make a quick casserole by stirring together 1 cup grain, chopped leftover veggies, chopped poultry, and hummus. Pour into a casserole dish and bake at 425°F for 25 minutes, until bubbly.

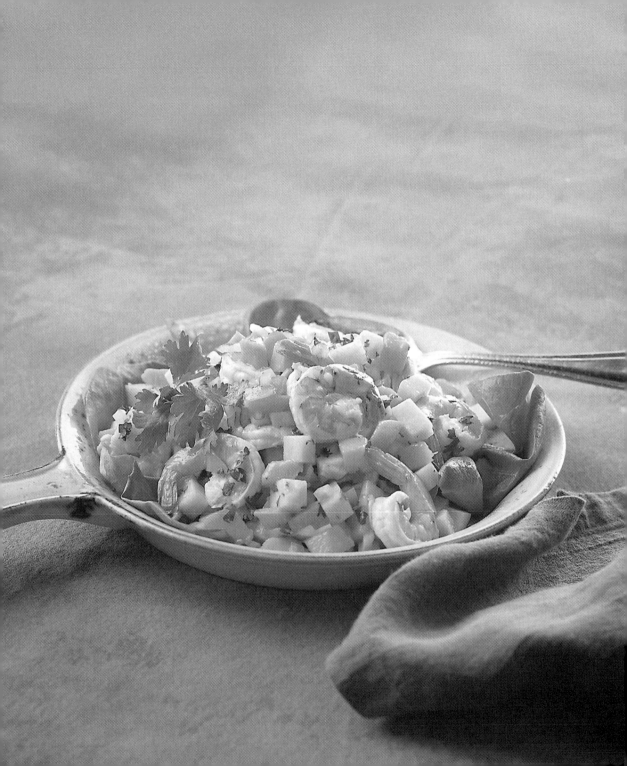

DINNER

For most of us, dinner is the big-deal meal of the day. We may skip breakfast and grab some random lunch food to wolf down or pick at while we toil at our desk, but dinner is different. Not only is it the one meal most of us plan for, it's likely the one meal we never miss. Dinner is a time to leave our stressful work and school day behind and decompress. With that in mind, I am going to use this chapter to challenge you to rethink dinner as a time to do something wonderful for yourself. That's something that superfood roots can help you with.

DINNER SALADS

CELERIAC LENTIL SALAD

MAKES 4–6 SERVINGS

Celeriac's subtle, earthy, celery-touched taste and gentle crunch make it a natural salad ingredient. In this high-protein dinner salad—which makes a perfect stand-alone supper—it pairs with lentils, fruit, and walnuts. This is a great way to get your antioxidants, fiber, and protein.

¼ cup walnut oil or extra virgin olive oil

⅓ cup apple cider vinegar

3 tablespoons honey

2 teaspoons ground cumin

2 teaspoons Dijon mustard

1 teaspoon salt

½ teaspoon pepper

3 cups cooked lentils, room temperature

3 cups water

1 teaspoon lemon juice or vinegar

1 medium celeriac, including the leafy top

1 Asian pear or large apple

2 shallots, minced

¼ chopped parsley, divided

¼ cup walnuts, roughly chopped

1. Whisk together the oil, vinegar, honey, cumin, mustard, salt, and pepper in a small bowl until completely combined. Set aside.

2. Place the cooked lentils in a large bowl.

3. In another large bowl, combine the water and lemon juice. Peel the celeriac (saving the leafy top) with a paring knife and cut into ⅛-inch slices, then cut those slices into long, thin matchsticks. As you cut pieces, immediately drop them into the water–lemon juice mixture. This will prevent them from turning brown.

4. Cut the pear the same way, into long matchsticks. Add to the bowl with the lentils.

5. Add the shallots to the bowl with the lentils.

6. Thinly slice the celeriac top and add to the bowl with the lentils.

7. Add ¼ cup of the chopped parsley to the bowl with the lentils.

8. Drain the celeriac and pat dry, if necessary. Add to the bowl with the lentils.

9. Drizzle the dressing over the lentil mixture. Gently toss to coat. Let sit for 20 minutes to allow the flavors to develop.

10. Taste and adjust the seasonings if necessary.

11. Garnish with the remaining ¼ cup of parsley and the walnuts.

GRILLED TUNA, TURNIP, AND RADISH SALAD

MAKES 4–6 SERVINGS

Adding an animal protein to a veggie-packed salad is a classic way to create a light meal. In this refreshing dish, grilled tuna teams up with turnips and radishes to create a heart-healthy meal that will leave you feeling full of energy.

- 4 tablespoons avocado oil or extra virgin olive oil, divided
- 4 cups sliced red onions (2 large onions)
- 2 teaspoons honey
- 1 tablespoon minced garlic
- ¼ cup red wine vinegar
- 2 tablespoons lime juice
- 2 teaspoons ground cumin
- ¼ cup chopped fresh cilantro

Salt and freshly ground pepper, to taste

- 2 small turnips, trimmed, peeled, and cut into matchsticks
- 1 bunch radishes, trimmed and sliced thin
- 2 seedless oranges
- 1 pound tuna steak or swordfish, about 1 inch thick
- 12 cups mesclun

1. Heat 2 tablespoons of the oil in a large sauté pan over medium-high heat. Add the onions and honey, and cook, stirring constantly, until well browned, 10–15 minutes. Add the garlic and cook for 1 minute more. Let cool to room temperature.

2. Transfer ¼ cup of the browned onions to a blender or food processor. Add the remaining 2 tablespoons of oil, vinegar, lime juice, and cumin, and puree until smooth. Add the cilantro and pulse to blend. Season with salt and pepper, and set aside.

3. Preheat the grill to medium-high.

4. Combine the turnips and radishes with the reserved onions in a large bowl.

5. With a sharp knife, remove the skin and white pith from the oranges and discard. (This is what it means to "supreme" an orange.)

6. Working over the large bowl to catch the juices, cut the orange segments from their surrounding membrane, letting the segments fall into the bowl with the turnip. Squeeze the juice from the membranes into the bowl. Season with salt and pepper.

7. Season both sides of tuna with salt and pepper. Grill over medium-high heat until just cooked through, 4–5 minutes per side. Let rest for 5 minutes before cutting into thin slices. Add the tuna to the turnip mixture.

8. Toss the lettuce with the reserved dressing in a large shallow bowl. Spoon the tuna mixture into the center of the greens and serve.

SOUTHWESTERN SALAD

MAKES 4–6 SERVINGS

I just realized that every superfood cookbook I've written—and even many of the personal cookbooks I've written for clients—contains at least one Southwestern-style salad that features black beans and quinoa. So here is a rooty version for this cookbook! Protein, fiber, omega-3 fatty acids, vitamins, minerals, phytonutrients—they're all here!

- 6 *cups chopped romaine lettuce*
- 2 *cups cooked red quinoa, chilled*
- 2 *cups cooked black beans*
- 1 *cup corn kernels (fresh or frozen)*
- 1 *small jicama, peeled and diced*
- 1 *small beet, trimmed, peeled, and grated*
- 2 *carrots, trimmed, peeled, and grated*
- 1 *small red pepper, chopped*
- ½ *red onion, diced*
- 1 *avocado, diced*
- ¼ *cup pepitas or sunflower seeds*
- 1 *14-ounce can coconut cream*
- ¼ *cup fresh lime juice*
- 1 *small garlic clove*
- 1 *teaspoon mustard*
- 1 *teaspoon cider vinegar*
- ¼ *cup finely chopped fresh cilantro*

Salt and pepper, to taste

1. Add the lettuce, quinoa, beans, corn, jicama, beet, carrots, red pepper, onion, avocado, and pepitas to a large bowl. Set aside without tossing.

2. Add the coconut cream, lime juice, garlic, mustard, vinegar, cilantro, salt, and pepper to a blender or food processor. Process until smooth.

3. Drizzle the amount of dressing that seems right for you over the salad ingredients. Toss to blend.

4. Refrigerate any extra dressing in a sealed container for up to 1 week.

TROPICAL SHRIMP SALAD WITH ROOTS

MAKES 4–6 SERVINGS

I don't eat shrimp very often, but when I do, I enjoy it paired with tropical flavors. This stand-alone salad is one of my favorites.

- 3 *tablespoons fresh lime juice*
- ¼ *cup fresh pineapple chunks*
- 6 *tablespoons coconut oil, avocado oil, or extra virgin olive oil, divided*

Salt and pepper, to taste

- 1 *pound uncooked large shrimp, peeled, deveined, and sliced in half lengthwise*
- 2 *tablespoons fresh lemon juice*
- 2 *large mangoes, peeled, pitted, and cut into ½-inch cubes (about 3 cups)*
- 2 *cups ½-inch cubes peeled jicama*
- 6 *radishes, trimmed and sliced thin*
- ½ *cup chopped red onion*
- 3 *tablespoons chopped fresh cilantro*

1. Add the lime juice and pineapple to a blender and process until smooth.

2. Pulse in 4 tablespoons of the oil and process until emulsified. Season with salt and pepper and set aside.

3. Heat the remaining 2 tablespoons of oil in a large sauté pan. Add the shrimp and lemon juice, salt and pepper to taste, and sauté just until the shrimp are cooked, 2–5 minutes. Set aside to cool, then refrigerate until ready to use. (You can do this step a day ahead if you'd like.)

4. In a large bowl, mix together the mangoes, jicama, radishes, onion, and cilantro.

5. When ready to serve, add shrimp to the mango-root mixture and toss with the pineapple dressing.

DINNER SOUPS AND STEWS

BARLEY-ROOT SOUP

MAKES 6 SERVINGS

This vegetarian soup is hearty, delicious, and so filled with fiber and antioxidants that I recommend enjoying it weekly. Feel free to play with the veggies a bit. If you don't have kale, use cabbage. If you don't have a carrot, try another parsnip. And so on.

8   *cups vegetable or beef broth*

½   *cup pearl barley*

1   *carrot, trimmed, peeled, and cut into ½-inch slices*

1   *celeriac, trimmed, peeled, and cut into ½-inch slices*

1   *parsnip, trimmed, peeled, cored, and cut into ½-inch slices*

1   *rutabaga, peeled and cut into ½-inch pieces*

1   *turnip, peeled and cut into ½-inch pieces*

1   *cup chopped kale or collards (or use turnip or rutabaga leaves)*

1   *onion, diced*

1   *15-ounce can diced tomatoes, with liquid*

1   *bay leaf*

1   *teaspoon salt*

½   *teaspoon dried sage*

½   *teaspoon dried thyme*

Pinch of freshly ground pepper

Pinch cayenne

1. Add the broth to a large soup pot over medium-high heat. Bring to a boil and add the barley.

2. Reduce the heat to medium-low, cover, and allow to simmer until the barley is tender, about 20 minutes.

3. Add the remaining ingredients. Turn the heat to medium-high and bring to a boil.

4. Reduce the heat to low, cover, and simmer until all the vegetables are tender, about 30 minutes.

5. Discard the bay leaf before serving.

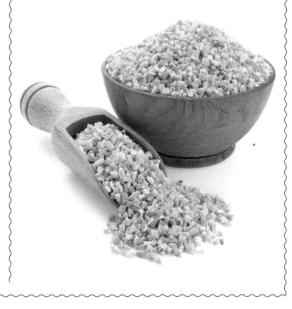

BEEF-AND-ROOT STEW

MAKES 8 SERVINGS

Protein, fiber, and plenty of antioxidant nutrients make this rooty take on a traditional stew a great stand-alone meal. Feel free to augment with a green salad if you'd like.

- ¼ cup extra virgin olive oil
- 2 pounds beef stew meat, cut in 1½-inch slices
- 3 cloves garlic, minced
- 1 shallot
- 1 medium onion, diced
- 2 cups red wine (or use beer or stout or more beef broth)
- 4 cups beef broth, plus more as needed
- 1 tablespoon Worcestershire sauce
- 2–3 tablespoons tomato paste
- ½ teaspoon paprika
- ½ teaspoon thyme
- ½ teaspoon allspice
- ½ teaspoon salt
- ½ teaspoon black pepper
- 2 red-flesh or blue potatoes, cut the same size or a bit smaller than the meat
- 2 carrots, roughly sliced
- 2 parsnips, roughly sliced
- 1 small turnip, roughly sliced
- 2 tablespoons tapioca starch (optional)
- Minced fresh parsley, for garnish

1. Heat the oil in a large soup pot or Dutch oven. Add the beef and brown on each side for 30 seconds (do not allow the meat to cook through!). Quickly remove the beef from the pan and place it in a single layer on a plate. Set the plate aside in the refrigerator.

2. Add the garlic, shallot, and onion to the pan and cook until softened, about 3 minutes. Pour in the wine, broth, Worcestershire sauce, tomato paste, paprika, thyme, allspice, salt, and pepper.

3. Return the beef to the pot. Cover and simmer on low heat until the meat is very tender, about 1½–2 hours. If the liquid level gets too low, add more broth as needed.

4. Add the potatoes, carrots, parsnips, and turnip and continue to simmer until the vegetables are tender and the liquid is reduced, about 30 minutes.

5. If you prefer your stew thicker, remove 1 cup of the cooking liquid. Whisk the tapioca starch into it, then add the mixture back to the stew pot and simmer for an additional 10 minutes.

6. Stir in the parsley.

7. Serve immediately or, preferably, allow to sit overnight to let the flavors develop.

SALMON-VEGGIE CHOWDER

MAKES 6 SERVINGS

This is a hearty, antioxidant-rich, dairy-free chowder that contains plenty of protein, fiber, and omega-3 fatty acids. If you enjoy salmon, you really must try this recipe. However, do not try this one if you don't have fresh dill—it is a required ingredient.

1   *tablespoon extra virgin oil*

1   *carrot, trimmed, peeled, and chopped*

1   *celery stalk, chopped*

1   *salsify, trimmed, peeled, and chopped*

1   *red-flesh potato, peeled and chopped*

5½ *cups chicken broth*

1   *12-ounce skinned salmon fillet, fresh or frozen*

2   *cups cauliflower florets, chopped*

3   *tablespoons chopped fresh chives*

2   *cups leftover mashed Yukon Gold (or other golden) potatoes*

¼   *cup chopped fresh dill*

1   *tablespoon Dijon mustard*

Salt and pepper, to taste

1. Heat the oil in a large saucepan or Dutch oven over medium heat. Add the carrot, celery, salsify, and red potato. Sauté until the vegetables just begin to brown, 3–4 minutes.

2. Add the broth, salmon, cauliflower, and chives and bring to a simmer. Cover and cook, maintaining a gentle simmer, until the salmon is just cooked through, 5–8 minutes. Remove the salmon to a cutting board. Flake into bite-size pieces with a fork.

3. Stir the leftover mashed potatoes, dill, and mustard into the soup until well blended.

4. Return to a simmer. Add the salmon and reheat. Season with salt and pepper.

SPICED ROOT DAL SOUP

MAKES 6 SERVINGS

I collect dal recipes. Some of my favorites come from clients. This one is an amalgamation of recipes shared by clients and dear friends Cindy Goodman, Ann Brosnan, and Jill Watson. Feel free to try different veggies in place of the ones I've listed below.

2   *tablespoons coconut oil*

2   *onions, minced*

2   *sweet potatoes, peeled and chopped*

2   *carrots, trimmed, peeled, and chopped*

2   *parsnips, trimmed, peeled, and chopped*

1   *jalapeño, minced*

1   *tablespoon ground cumin*

½   *tablespoon Madras curry powder*

1   *cup dried red lentils*

5   *cups vegetable broth*

1   *15-ounce can coconut milk*

Salt and pepper, to taste

3   *tablespoons cilantro leaves, roughly chopped*

1. Heat the oil in a large saucepan over medium heat. Sauté the onions until softened, about 5 minutes.

2. Add the sweet potatoes, carrots, and parsnips and cook for another 5 minutes.

3. Add the jalapeño, cumin, and curry powder and cook for another 2 minutes.

4. Add the lentils and vegetable broth to the pot and bring to a boil.

5. Lower the heat, stir in the coconut milk, and allow the soup to simmer until the lentils are soft, about 20 minutes.

6. Season with salt and pepper to taste and stir in the cilantro. You can serve the soup immediately, but I think it tastes best the next day, after being given a day to let the flavors develop.

STARCHY SIDES

BARLEY BAKE

MAKES 6 SERVINGS

Barley is a lovely, chewy grain. Kids love it—or at least mine do. So does my picky husband. This makes me happy because I know that just one serving of the stuff gives him more than 128 percent of the daily requirement for fiber, 36 percent for iron, 30 percent for vitamin B6, and 61 percent for magnesium. And in this dish he also gets all the phytonutrients in the salsify and sweet potato. **NOTE:** Barley does contain some gluten, so if you have celiac disease, try this recipe with brown, red, or black rice.

¼ cup extra virgin olive oil

1 medium onion, diced

1 shallot, minced

1 cup uncooked pearl barley

½ cup pecans, roughly chopped

1 salsify, scorzonera, or burdock root, trimmed, peeled, and diced

1 sweet potato, peeled and diced

½ cup chopped fresh parsley

Salt and pepper, to taste

3 cups vegetable broth

1. Preheat the oven to 350°F.

2. Add the oil to a large sauté pan and heat over medium-high heat. Stir in the onion, shallot, barley, and pecans and cook until the barley is lightly browned, about 4 minutes.

3. Add the salsify, sweet potato, and parsley and sauté for about 2 more minutes. Season with salt and pepper.

4. Transfer the mixture to a 2-quart casserole dish and stir in the vegetable broth.

5. Bake 1 hour and 15 minutes, or until the liquid has been absorbed and the barley is tender.

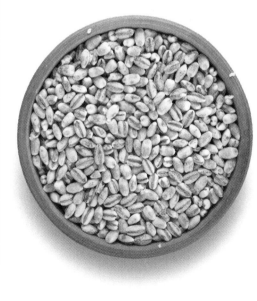

MILLET-ROOT PILAF

MAKES 4 SERVINGS

I am a millet fan. A serving of this seed will give you fiber, iron, vitamin B6, and magnesium. In this yummy recipe, you get all *that* goodness, *plus* the antioxidant benefits of root vegetables.

- *3 cups root vegetables of your choice, trimmed, peeled, and diced*
- *2 tablespoons extra virgin olive oil*
- *Salt and pepper, to taste*
- *1 cup uncooked millet*
- *2 cups of chicken or vegetable broth*
- *1 cup mixed fresh herbs, such as chives, cilantro, basil, parsley, dill, etc.*

1. Preheat the oven to 350°F.

2. Add the vegetables to a large bowl and toss them with the oil, salt, and pepper.

3. Transfer the vegetables to two baking sheets, arranging them in a single layer, being careful not to crowd them.

4. Bake for 15–20 minutes, or until they begin to caramelize.

5. While the vegetables cook, place a medium saucepan over medium-high heat. When the pan is hot, add the millet and dry-toast it until it begins popping.

6. Add the broth to the pan and season with a generous amount of salt and pepper (millet is very bland and needs a lot of salt).

7. Bring the pot to a boil, then reduce the heat to low, cover, and simmer for about 15 minutes, or until the liquid is absorbed. Do not uncover or stir while it cooks! This will lead to mushy millet.

8. When the millet is done, remove it from the heat and let sit for about 10 minutes.

9. Turn the millet out into a serving bowl, add the herbs, adjust the seasoning, and fluff the grain gently with a fork.

10. Gently fold in the roasted vegetables and serve.

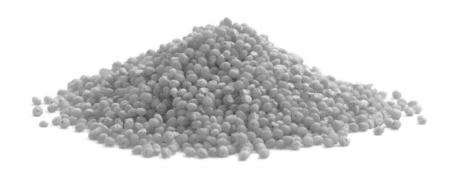

MOROCCAN QUINOA WITH ROOTS

MAKES 4 SERVINGS

Quinoa has a delicate crunch that people love. It also contains colossal amounts of nutrients, including 8 grams of protein per serving and large amounts of manganese, magnesium, folate, zinc, omega-3 fatty acids, and a host of anti-inflammatory phytonutrients. Add that to root vegetables, which have their own phytonutrients, and wow, this recipe is good for you!

3 *parsnips, trimmed, peeled, and cut into ½-inch pieces*

2 *carrots, trimmed, peeled, and cut into ½-inch pieces*

6 *tablespoons extra virgin olive oil, divided*

1 *tablespoon ground cumin*

2 *teaspoons ground turmeric*

1 *teaspoon ground cinnamon*

Salt and pepper, to taste

2 *cups vegetable or chicken broth*

1 *cup uncooked quinoa, rinsed*

¼ *cup slivered almonds*

2 *tablespoons parsley*

1. Preheat the oven to 400°F.

2. Add the parsnips and carrots to a large bowl and toss with 2 tablespoons of the oil, the cumin, turmeric, and cinnamon. Spread the vegetables in a single layer on two baking sheets, making sure not to crowd them, and season generously with salt and pepper.

3. Roast, stirring once, until the vegetables are caramelized, about 35 minutes. Remove from the oven and set aside to cool.

4. While the vegetables are roasting, add the broth to a saucepan over high heat. Bring to a boil and add the quinoa.

5. Reduce the heat to low, cover the quinoa, and allow to simmer until the quinoa is cooked and the broth absorbed, about 10–15 minutes.

6. Transfer the quinoa to a large bowl and gently fold in the roasted vegetables, almonds, and parsley.

7. Gently stir in the remaining 4 tablespoons of olive oil, season with salt and pepper, and serve.

SMASHED PURPLE POTATOES

MAKES 4 SERVINGS

For a while in the early 2000s, it seemed as if every restaurant in Manhattan had smashed potatoes on their menu. Which was fine by me—I love these things! This version, made with purple potatoes, satisfies your potato craving while also providing large amounts of fiber and antioxidants. Feel free to sub in red-flesh or golden potatoes.

1 *pound baby purple potatoes, skins on*

4 *tablespoons extra virgin olive oil*

Salt and pepper, to taste

2 *tablespoons parsley, chopped*

1. In a large pot, cook the potatoes with skins on in heavily salted boiling water until tender, approximately 15 minutes.

2. Remove the potatoes from the pot and allow them to cool.

3. Heat the oil in a large pan over high heat. Add the potatoes, making sure not to crowd the pan (you can work in batches, if necessary). Allow the potatoes to fry for 1 minute in the hot oil, then, using the bottom of a heavy glass, smash each one slightly, so they look like croquettes.

4. Let them continue to fry for 5 minutes, or until crispy. Feel free to flip them if you want two crispy sides, or enjoy them as-is.

5. Season with salt and pepper and sprinkle with parsley before serving.

WHAT TO DO WITH LEFTOVER COOKED POTATOES

- Refry them. Yum!
- Mash them with a bit of hot milk, salt, pepper, and your favorite seasonings.
- Add to a pot of stew or chili.
- Roughly chop and add to a frying pan with a couple of tablespoons oil, minced onion, and perhaps some shredded beef or chicken. Sauté until brown for a quick hash.
- Cook in a bit of oil and curry powder for fast Indian-style potatoes. Add 1 can chickpeas if you'd like some protein.
- If you make your own bread, knead ½ cup peeled cooked potato into your next dough. This not only improves the dough's pliability, it increases the finished product's "keepability."

VEGGIE SIDES

CARROT-HAZELNUT PUREE

MAKES 4 SERVINGS

This recipe is a cooking school staple. Carrots are cooked and pureed with seasonings to create an elegant, nutrient-rich side dish. If you have any of this left over, you can thin it with a bit of broth for a delicious soup.

- 1 *pound carrots (5–6 medium), cut into ½-inch pieces*
- 2 *medium red-flesh potatoes, peeled and cut into ½-inch pieces*
- 1 *tablespoon extra virgin olive oil*
- 1 *shallot, minced*
- 2 *tablespoons chopped hazelnuts, toasted*
- 2 *teaspoons freshly grated orange zest*
- 1 *small clove garlic, minced*
- 2 *teaspoons hazelnut oil or extra virgin olive oil*

Salt and pepper, to taste

1. Bring 1 inch of water to a boil in a large saucepan or Dutch oven fitted with a steamer basket. Steam the carrots and potatoes until very soft, 12–15 minutes. Set aside.

2. Add the oil, shallots, and hazelnuts to a sauté pan over medium-high heat and sauté until the shallots are soft, about 3 minutes.

3. Add the carrots, potatoes, shallots, and hazelnuts to the bowl of a food processor and pulse a few times to blend.

4. Add the orange zest, garlic, hazelnut oil, salt, and pepper. Process until smooth.

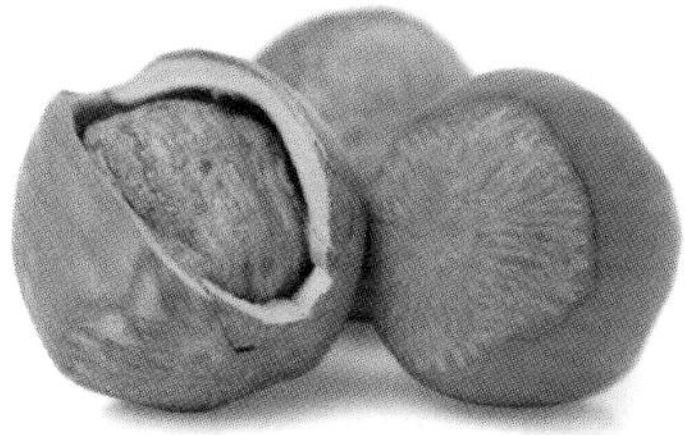

ROASTED ROOT VEGETABLES

MAKES 8 SERVINGS

Everyone needs a good roasted root veggie recipe, and this is mine. Well, it's really more of a blueprint than a recipe—feel free to substitute other veggies (even of the non-root variety) for the ones I've listed here. I make one or more pans of this every week and enjoy it as a side dish, as well as add roasted veggies to salads, wraps, grain salads, and so on.

1 *purple or red-flesh potatoes, unpeeled, scrubbed, and cut into 1-inch pieces*

1 *pound celeriac, trimmed, peeled, and cut into 1-inch pieces*

1 *pound rutabagas, trimmed, peeled, and cut into 1-inch pieces*

1 *pound carrots, trimmed, peeled, and cut into 1-inch pieces*

1 *pound parsnips, trimmed, peeled, and cut into 1-inch pieces*

1 *pound sunchokes, cut into 1-inch pieces*

2 *onions, cut into 1-inch pieces*

1 *leek (optional) cut into 1-inch pieces*

2 *tablespoons chopped fresh rosemary*

⅓ *cup extra virgin olive oil*

10 *garlic cloves, peeled*

Salt and pepper, to taste

1. Preheat the oven to 400°F.

2. Combine all ingredients in a large bowl and toss to combine. Be generous with the salt and pepper.

3. Divide the vegetable mixture between two or three shallow baking pans, making sure not to crowd them.

4. Roast 30 minutes, then rotate the baking sheets (in case your oven heat is uneven), giving the veggies in each pan a stir.

5. Continue to roast until all vegetables are caramelized, about 30 additional minutes.

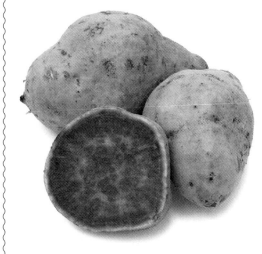

SAUTÉ OF ROOT VEGETABLES

MAKES 8 SERVINGS

I love sautéing vegetables. They take on a fork-tender texture and lovely sweetness when cooked on the stovetop in a bit of good oil. This is another one of my favorite ways to enjoy root veggies. It comes together very quickly, making it a fast side dish. Toss in some chickpeas or leftover chicken, pork, or beef for a simple meal. Oh, and yes, of course you can substitute other roots for the ones below!

3 *tablespoons extra virgin olive oil*

3 *medium carrots, trimmed and cut into matchsticks*

3 *leeks, white and light green part only, cut into matchsticks*

½ *large rutabaga, trimmed, peeled, and cut into matchsticks*

1 *celeriac, trimmed, peeled, and cut into matchsticks*

1 *cup vegetable or chicken broth*

1 *tablespoon chopped fresh thyme*

Salt and pepper, to taste

1. Add the oil to a large sauté pan over medium heat. Stir in the carrots, leeks, rutabaga, and celeriac, and sauté until softened, about 3–5 minutes.

2. Add the broth and thyme and bring to a simmer.

3. Reduce the heat to low, cover, and cook, stirring occasionally, until the vegetables are tender and the broth has evaporated, 10–15 minutes.

4. Season with salt and pepper.

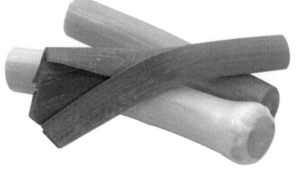

TURKISH CELERIAC

MAKES 6 SERVINGS

This refreshing, easy recipe hails from Turkey, where it is a popular side dish. It is a lovely introduction to this nutritious root. If your celeriac comes with stalks attached, save them to use in place of the celery. If you have a nice vegetable or chicken broth you'd like to use, go ahead and use it in place of the water.

2   large celeriac roots, trimmed and peeled

Juice of ½ lemon

Juice of 1 orange

1   large carrot, trimmed, peeled, and sliced

1   small onion

2   celery stalks (or use the stalks from the celeriac)

1   teaspoon salt

¼   teaspoon black pepper

1   teaspoon honey or raw sugar

½   cup extra virgin olive oil, divided

1. Peel the celeriac and slice into ½-inch slices. Place them in the bottom of a large nonreactive saucepan.

2. Quickly cover the celeriac with the lemon and orange juices. In addition to flavoring the dish, the citrus juice will help keep the celeriac from browning.

3. Arrange the carrot slices on top of the celeriac.

4. Peel the onion and cut it in quarters. Coarsely slice each quarter and separate the rings. Arrange the rings of onions on top of the carrots.

5. Coarsely chop the celery (or celeriac stalks) and layer them on top of the onions.

6. Sprinkle the salt, pepper, and honey over the celery, then drizzle on ¼ cup of the olive oil.

7. Add about ½ cup water. Turn the heat on high and bring the pan to a boil.

8. Reduce the heat to low, cover the pan, and let the vegetables simmer until tender and the liquid is reduced. (Add more water if needed.)

9. Gently remove the vegetables from the pan and arrange them on a serving plate. Drizzle the remaining ¼ cup of olive oil over the top.

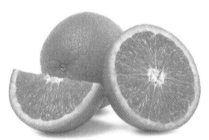

ENTREES

ROAST CHICKEN AND ROOT VEGETABLES WITH MUSTARD-ROSEMARY SAUCE

MAKES 6 SERVINGS

Everyone needs a good roast chicken recipe. If you don't have one you love, let me suggest this one. It comes with a healthy amount of nutrient-dense root veggies and a scrumptious mustard sauce. Enjoy!

⅓ *cup whole-grain mustard*

⅓ *cup extra virgin olive oil, plus extra for the baking pans*

2½ *tablespoons chopped fresh rosemary*

Salt and pepper, to taste

1 *4-pound roasting chicken, rinsed, patted dry, and giblets removed*

2 *large red onions, each cut into 8 wedges, peeled*

2 *blue potatoes, cut into 1½-inch pieces*

1½ *pounds rutabaga or turnips, cut into 1½-inch pieces*

1 *pound peeled baby carrots*

1 *cup chicken broth*

1. Preheat the oven to 375°F.

2. Whisk the mustard, oil, rosemary, salt, and pepper in bowl.

3. Place the chicken in large roasting pan and brush with half of the mustard mixture. Roast until a thermometer inserted into the thickest part of the thigh registers 170°F, about 1 hour 45 minutes. When cooked, remove from the oven and set aside to cool.

4. Meanwhile, add the onions, potatoes, rutabaga, and carrots to a large bowl and toss with 1 tablespoon of the reserved mustard sauce.

5. Rub a bit of oil onto two baking pans. Place the vegetables in a single layer on the baking pans, being careful not to crowd them. Roast until they begin to caramelize, about 50 minutes, stirring about halfway through.

6. Skim the fat from the juices in the pan with the chicken; discard or save for another use. Add the pan juices to a saucepan and cook over medium-high heat until the mixture is reduced to about 1¼ cups, about 5–8 minutes.

7. Season the sauce with salt and pepper and decant into a gravy boat.

8. Arrange the chicken on a serving platter, surrounded by vegetables. Pass the sauce separately.

BRAISED BRISKET AND ROOTS

MAKES 8 SERVINGS

Roots are natural companions to roasted meats of all kinds. In this brisket recipe, a large number of roots cook alongside the meat, creating a savory meal. Feel free to use other roots if you'd like. **NOTE:** The recipe seems long, but it does come together quickly.

1   tablespoon extra virgin olive oil

2   pounds flat, first-cut brisket, trimmed

3   medium onions, sliced into half-moons

¼   teaspoon allspice

2   teaspoons chopped fresh thyme, or ¾ teaspoon dried

1   teaspoon sweet paprika

½   teaspoon salt

½   teaspoon freshly ground pepper

2   bay leaves

1   cup dry white wine

3   cups reduced-sodium beef broth

3   medium carrots, peeled

2   medium parsnips, peeled and cored

2   burdock, salsify, or scorzonera roots, trimmed and peeled

1   medium rutabaga (about ¾ pound), peeled

1   teaspoon Dijon mustard

2   teaspoons tapioca starch or arrowroot, or 1 tablespoon cornstarch

1. Preheat the oven to 325°F.

2. Heat the oil in a large ovenproof saucepot or Dutch oven over medium-high heat. Add the brisket and brown on both sides, about 3 minutes per side. Transfer to a large platter and set aside.

3. Add the onions to the pot and cook, stirring frequently, until softened, about 2 minutes.

4. Stir in the allspice, thyme, paprika, salt, pepper, and bay leaves, then pour in the wine. Bring to a boil and cook for 3 minutes.

5. Stir in the broth and return the brisket to the pot along with any accumulated juices. Bring to a simmer.

6. Cover the pot and place in the oven. Bake for 1½ hours.

7. Meanwhile, cut the carrots, parsnips, burdock, and rutabaga into 2×½×½-inch sticks.

8. Open the oven, take the cover off the brisket, and stir the mustard and tapioca starch into the juices in the pan, using a fork to whisk them into the liquid.

9. Tuck the sliced vegetables around the meat, spooning a bit of the meat juices over them.

10. Put the lid back on the pot and bake for 45–60 minutes more, or until the vegetables are soft and the meat is done.

11. Remove the pot carefully from the oven, remove the lid, and let rest for 45–90 minutes at room temperature.

12. Transfer the meat to a cutting board and slice it against the grain. Transfer it to a large serving platter and mound the veggies around it. Spoon the pot juices over the meat, or decant to a gravy boat and pass separately.

13. If you'd like a thicker sauce, place it in a saucepan over medium-high heat and reduce.

ROOT VEGETABLE CURRY

MAKES 6 SERVINGS

Most of my meals are vegan, so I am always on the lookout for high-protein, easy-to-make, economical dishes that don't use a lot of exotic ingredients. This is one of my go-to recipes. I serve it with quinoa or millet, but feel free to pair it with any grain you'd like.

2   *tablespoons coconut oil*

1   *onion, chopped*

1½ *tablespoons grated fresh ginger*

1   *teaspoon ground cumin*

1   *medium-size purple potato, diced*

1   *medium-size sweet potato, diced*

1   *turnip, peeled and diced*

1   *parsnip, peeled and diced*

1   *garlic clove, minced*

½   *jalapeño, minced*

1   *teaspoon turmeric*

1   *teaspoon ground coriander*

2   *cups cooked chickpeas*

1   *14-ounce can coconut milk, divided*

Salt, to taste

¼   *cup cilantro leaves, chopped*

¼   *cup Thai basil or 2 tablespoons chopped regular basil leaves with 2 tablespoons chopped mint leaves (optional, but amazing)*

1. Heat the oil in a large skillet over medium heat. Cook the onion, ginger, and cumin until the onion begins to soften and turn translucent, about 3 minutes.

2. Add the purple potato, sweet potato, turnip, parsnip, garlic, jalapeño, turmeric, coriander, and chickpeas and sauté about 8 minutes. Add ¼ cup of the coconut milk. Continue cooking for a couple of minutes, allowing the coconut milk to evaporate.

3. Add an additional ¼ cup of the coconut milk. Continue to cook about 5 minutes, or until the veggies are just al dente.

4. Add the remaining coconut milk, salt to taste, then add the cilantro and basil (if using). Allow the mixture to come to a simmer and cook an additional 2–3 minutes before removing from the heat.

SALMON ON A BED OF ROOTY LENTILS

MAKES 4 SERVINGS

I use a lot of lentils in my cooking. They are full of protein and fiber, they are economical, and they cook quickly. Here, the green Le Puy lentils (which hold their shape so beautifully) are paired with root veggies and salmon. This is a nutritionist's dream meal!

- 2 teaspoons extra virgin olive oil
- 1 shallot, minced
- 1 garlic clove, minced
- 2 cups chicken broth, plus more if needed
- ½ cup dry white wine, or additional broth
- 1 cup uncooked green lentils
- 1½ teaspoons chopped fresh thyme, or ½ teaspoon dried
- ¼ teaspoon salt
- Pepper, to taste
- 2 carrots, trimmed, peeled, and diced
- 2 small turnips, trimmed, peeled, and diced
- 1 pound fresh or frozen salmon fillet, skin removed, cut into 4 portions
- 2 tablespoons chopped fresh parsley

1. Heat the oil in a large sauté pan or Dutch oven over medium heat. Sauté the shallots and garlic for about 30 seconds.

2. Add the broth, wine, lentils, thyme, salt, and pepper and bring to a boil.

3. Reduce the heat to low and simmer, covered, until the lentils just start to get tender, about 25 minutes.

4. Add the carrots and turnips, and simmer until the vegetables are tender, about 10 minutes more, adding more broth if necessary.

5. Taste and adjust the seasonings. Lay the salmon fillets on top, cover the pan, and cook until the salmon is opaque in the center, 8–10 minutes.

6. Remove the salmon from the top of the lentils, ladle the lentils and vegetables into shallow bowls, and top with the salmon. Sprinkle parsley over each serving.

VEGAN SHEPHERD'S PIE

MAKES 6 SERVINGS

I love shepherd's pie, be it vegetarian or meat-filled! The nice thing about this vegan dish is that it's a great way to enjoy a range of nutritious roots. **NOTE:** There are a number of steps to this dish, but don't despair. The dish comes together very easily. Really!

- 2½ pounds (about 4 large) gold potatoes, peeled and quartered
- 6 parsnips, trimmed, peeled, and roughly chopped
- 1 cup coconut milk or coconut cream (with a 14-ounce can, you will have leftover milk or cream; save for another recipe)

4 tablespoons extra virgin olive oil, divided

Salt and pepper, to taste

1½ cups uncooked brown or green lentils

4 cups vegetable broth, divided

1 large onion, diced

2–3 cloves garlic, minced

2 large carrots or 1 sweet potato, peeled, trimmed, and diced

½ celeriac, trimmed, diced, and brushed with lemon juice to keep it from browning

6 ounces mushrooms of your choice, sliced

1 can tomato paste

1 teaspoon dried rosemary

¼ teaspoon dried thyme

1 teaspoon paprika, plus more for garnish

¼ teaspoon cayenne

1. Place the potatoes and parsnips in a large pot of cool, generously salted water over high heat. Bring to a boil, cover, and simmer until the vegetables are fork-tender, about 30 minutes.

2. Drain and return the potatoes and parsnips to the pot with the coconut cream, 2 tablespoons of the oil, salt, and pepper. Mash with a potato masher until smooth. Set aside.

3. While the potatoes are cooking, add the lentils and 3½ cups of the broth to a saucepan over medium-high heat and bring to a boil. Reduce the heat to low, cover the pot, and simmer until the lentils have absorbed all the liquid and are soft, about 30–35 minutes. Set the lentils aside.

4. Heat the remaining 2 tablespoons of olive oil in a large sauté pan over medium heat. Add the onion and garlic and cook until the onion is translucent and begins to caramelize, about 10 minutes.

5. Add the carrots and celeriac and cook until tender, about 7 minutes.

6. Add the mushrooms and cook another 3 minutes.

7. Add the tomato paste, rosemary, thyme, paprika, and cayenne and ½ cup of the remaining broth. You want a relatively dry mixture, so simmer until the liquid is reduced. Taste and adjust the salt and pepper.

8. Preheat the oven to 350°F.

9. Mix the lentils and vegetables together and transfer to a large casserole dish. Top with the mashed potato-parsnip mixture, spreading it delicately to completely cover the lentils.

10. Sprinkle with extra paprika, if desired.

11. Bake for 20 minutes, or until bubbly.

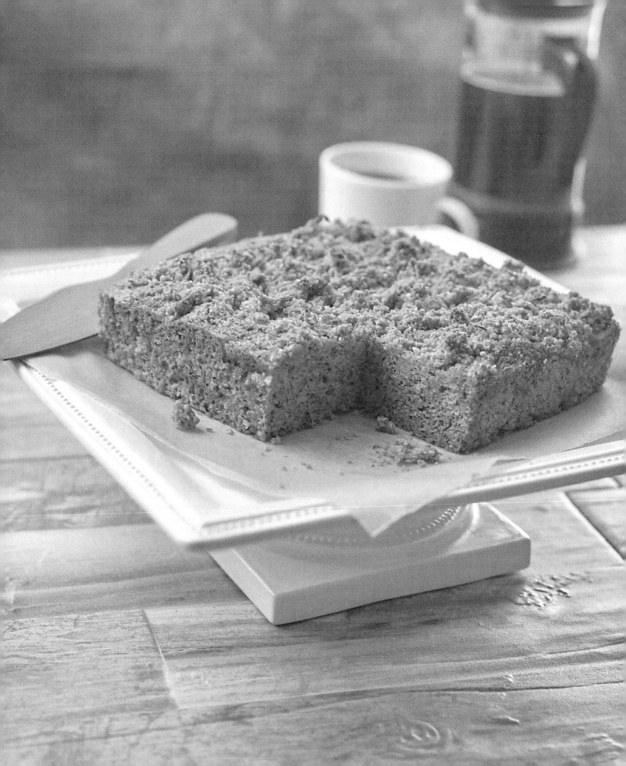

DESSERTS

Root vegetables—they just make you think about dessert, don't they? Kidding! Outside of overly sweet carrot cake and ubiquitous sweet potato pie, roots don't make frequent appearances in modern desserts. It wasn't always that way, however. There was a time when parsnips, rutabagas, turnips, and beets made regular appearances in after-meal sweets. It makes sense, considering how naturally sweet most roots are. While I am not a proponent of eating more desserts, I would like to use this chapter's well-curated collection of recipes to show you some delicious ways to sneak more roots into your life. Based on superfood ingredients, these treats make the most of the natural sweetness of roots and their ability to improve your health. Enjoy!

CAKES, CUPCAKES, AND BARS

BEET CAKE

MAKES 12 SERVINGS

You may have tasted a chocolate beet cake before—the recipes are quite popular on the Internet—but this pink beauty is vanilla-based, so there is nothing to hide its bright color. Feel free to use golden beets if you'd like, for a subtler look. Eat it as-is, or try it with Coconut Cream Frosting (page 150).

4 eggs

2 cups coconut sugar (pulse a few times in a food processor to make it fine) or cane sugar

1 cup coconut oil

2 cups whole-wheat pastry flour

2 teaspoons baking powder

1½ teaspoons baking soda

1 teaspoon cinnamon

½ teaspoon allspice

2 teaspoons vanilla

3 cups shredded fresh beets

1. Preheat the oven to 350°F.

2. Grease and flour a 9-inch Bundt pan. (Alternatively, you can use two 9-inch round pans or a 9×13-inch baking pan, or make 24 cupcakes.)

3. In the bowl of a stand mixer fitted with a paddle attachment, beat together the eggs, sugar, and oil until light and fluffy.

4. In a separate bowl, whisk together the flour, baking powder, baking soda, cinnamon, and allspice.

5. Add the flour mixture to the egg mixture and mix well.

6. Add the vanilla and beets and mix for an additional minute to combine.

7. Pour into a prepared pan and bake for 45 minutes, or until a toothpick inserted in the center comes out clean. (Adjust the cooking time as necessary if you're using a different pan.)

WORKING WITH COCONUT SUGAR

Coconut sugar is the dried sap of the coconut tree. Many nutritionists prefer it to cane sugar because—while still a sweetener that should be enjoyed in moderation—1 teaspoon of coconut sugar contains 15 calories and 4 carbohydrates, as opposed to cane sugar's 16 calories and 5 carbohydrates.

In most recipes—including baked goods—coconut can be used cup-for-cup in place of table sugar. However, because it is much coarser than regular table sugar, it can affect the quality of your recipes. For that reason, when I bake with coconut sugar, I always pulse it a few times in a clean coffee grinder or in my food processor to create a fine-grained finish. I suggest you do the same.

GLUTEN-FREE SPICED PARSNIP CUPCAKES

MAKES 12 CUPCAKES

This recipe is gluten-free. Parsnips add moisture and keeping quality, as well as a lilting sweetness.

¾ cup rice flour

1 cup oat flour

2 tablespoons tapioca starch

2 teaspoons baking powder

1 teaspoon cinnamon

½ teaspoon vanilla powder

½ teaspoon ground ginger

Pinch of cloves

Pinch of salt

4 eggs

¾ cup honey, coconut nectar, or maple syrup, amber or dark

¾ cup coconut oil

3 medium parsnips, trimmed, peeled, and grated

Zest of 1 orange

1. Preheat the oven to 350°F.

2. Line a muffin tin with 12 paper baking cups. Set aside.

3. In a large bowl, whisk together the flours, tapioca starch, baking powder, cinnamon, vanilla powder, ginger, cloves, and salt. Set aside.

4. Add the eggs to the bowl of a stand mixer fitted with a paddle attachment. Beat on medium-high speed until frothy.

5. Add in honey and oil and beat for another two minutes.

6. Add the parsnip and orange zest and beat just until blended.

7. Add the flour mixture and beat 1 more minute.

8. Distribute the mixture evenly into the baking cups and bake for about 20 minutes, or until the cupcakes are firm to the touch. Allow to cool for 1 hour in the tin before handling.

HEALTHIER CARROT CAKE

MAKES 12 SERVINGS

I am crazy for carrot cake—even though it is often filled with a ton of sugar and cheap cooking oil. This recipe, however, uses applesauce as a sweetener and relies on health-supportive coconut oil. I think you're going to like this! Frost it with Coconut Cream Frosting (page 150) or enjoy it plain as a snack cake.

2   *cups whole-wheat pastry flour*

1   *teaspoon baking soda*

1½ *teaspoons baking powder*

½   *teaspoon salt*

1½ *teaspoons cinnamon*

4   *large eggs*

1   *cup honey*

½   *cup coconut oil, plus more for the cake pans*

2   *teaspoon vanilla*

1   *cup applesauce, pear sauce, or pureed banana, sweet potato, or pumpkin*

3   *cups carrots, trimmed, peeled, and grated*

1. Preheat the oven to 350°F.

2. Grease and flour two 9-inch round or square cake pans.

3. In a medium bowl, whisk together the flour, baking soda, baking powder, salt, and cinnamon.

4. In the bowl of a stand mixer fitted with a paddle attachment, beat the eggs on medium-high speed until foamy.

5. Add in the honey and beat for another 5 minutes.

6. Add the oil, vanilla, and applesauce and beat for another 5 minutes.

7. Add the flour mixture ½ cup at a time, mixing on medium speed after each addition, until just incorporated.

8. Add the grated carrots and mix until just combined.

9. Divide the batter equally among the two cake pans and bake 28–30 minutes, or until a toothpick inserted in the center comes out clean.

10. Cool completely before removing from the pans.

PARSNIP SNACK CAKE

MAKES 10 SERVINGS

Parsnip cakes are a bit like carrot cakes, only with a deeper, more intriguing flavor and less sweetness. This version uses maple syrup as a sweetener and features orange juice and apples.

- ¾ cup liquid coconut oil
- ¾ cup coconut sugar or brown sugar
- ½ cup maple syrup, amber or dark
- 3 large eggs
- 2 cups all-purpose flour
- 2 teaspoons baking powder
- 2 teaspoons pumpkin pie spice
- 2 large or 4 medium parsnips, trimmed, peeled, and grated (3 cups)
- 1 medium apple (any variety), peeled, cored, and grated
- ½ cup pecans or hazelnuts, roughly chopped
- 1 tablespoon finely grated orange zest, preferably organic
- ⅓ cup fresh orange juice

1. Preheat the oven to 350°F.

2. Lightly grease and flour one 9×13-inch cake pan (or two 9-inch round pans).

3. Warm the oil, sugar, and maple syrup in a saucepan over low heat, stirring occasionally, until completely combined. Remove from the heat and let cool slightly.

4. In the bowl of a stand mixer fitted with a paddle attachment, beat the eggs on medium until blended, about 3 minutes.

5. Pour in the cooled oil-sugar mixture and beat for 3 minutes.

6. In a large bowl, whisk together the flour, baking powder, and pumpkin pie spice. Add to the mixing bowl and mix on medium speed until just mixed.

7. Add the parsnips, apple, nuts, orange zest, and orange juice to the bowl and mix until just combined.

8. Scrape the mixture into the prepared baking pan and bake for 30 minutes, or until a toothpick inserted in the center comes out clean.

9. Allow the cake to cool before cutting.

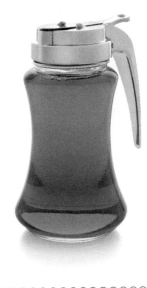

RUTABAGA BARS

MAKES 9 SERVINGS

A cross between cakey blondies and a snack cake, this yummy recipe features outrageously nutritious rutabaga. For a gluten-free recipe, you can use your favorite gluten-free all-purpose flour.

6 *large eggs*

2½ *cups coconut sugar or cane sugar*

1¼ *cup liquid coconut oil, plus more for greasing the pan*

2 *teaspoons vanilla*

2½ *cups all-purpose gluten-free flour*

2 *teaspoons baking powder*

2 *teaspoons baking soda*

¼ *teaspoon salt*

2 *teaspoons cinnamon*

1½ *cups grated rutabaga*

1. Heat the oven to 350°F.

2. Grease and flour a 9×9-inch baking pan

3. Add the eggs and sugar to the bowl of a stand mixer fitted with a paddle attachment. Beat on medium-high until frothy and pale in color.

4. Add the oil and vanilla and mix to blend.

5. In a separate large bowl, whisk together the flour, baking powder, baking soda, salt, and cinnamon. Dump into the mixing bowl and beat just to combine.

6. Add the rutabaga and mix on low just until combined.

7. Pour the mixture into the prepared pan and bake for 40 minutes, or until springy to the touch.

8. Allow to cool for 1 hour before cutting.

COCONUT CREAM FROSTING

1 *14-ounce can coconut cream, cold (chill overnight in the fridge)*

⅓ *cup coconut sugar or maple sugar, whirred in a clean coffee grinder or food processor to make it fine*

1 *teaspoon vanilla extract or other flavoring*

Add all ingredients to the mixing bowl of a stand mixer fitted with a whisk attachment. Beat until the ingredients are combined and the texture is smooth and fluffy.

PIES AND TARTS

CARROT PIE

MAKES 8 SERVINGS

Once upon a time, pies made with a variety of root vegetables were popular—including this scrumptious, antioxidant-rich carrot pie. I think it's a time we revisited using root vegetables in pies!

1   pound carrots, trimmed, peeled, and roughly chopped

½   cup honey

½   cup coconut sugar or brown sugar

1   cup coconut cream

½   tablespoon vanilla

¼   teaspoon salt

2   teaspoons five-spice powder, pumpkin pie spice, or apple pie spice

3   large eggs

1   9-inch prebaked pie shell of your choice

1. Preheat the oven to 350°F.

2. In a medium saucepan with a steamer insert, steam the carrots until very soft (or simply simmer in the smallest amount of water possible), about 15 minutes.

3. Transfer the carrots to a food processor and process until chunky.

4. Add the honey, sugar, coconut cream, vanilla, salt, five-spice powder, and eggs and process until smooth.

5. Pour into the prebaked pie shell and bake for 45 minutes, or until the custard is puffed on the edges and set in the middle.

6. Allow the pie to cool for 1 hour or more before slicing. This helps develop the flavors and firms up the pie.

WHIPPED COCONUT TOPPING

1   14-ounce can coconut cream (make sure it does not contain guar gum)

2   tablespoons powdered sugar

1   teaspoon tapioca starch

1. Set the can of coconut cream in the fridge for at least 1 hour, but preferably overnight.

2. Combine the cream, powdered sugar, and tapioca starch in a large bowl. Using electric beaters, beat the mixture for 2–3 minutes. It won't form stiff peaks like whipped dairy cream, but it will be stiff enough to dollop.

PARSNIP TART

MAKES 8 SERVINGS

This intriguing tart may remind you of a pumpkin pie, but it isn't quite as sweet. And there's something about it that you may not be able to place: The parsnip! I encourage you to give this old-fashioned tart a try.

- 2 *pounds medium parsnips, peeled, cored, and cut into large chunks*
- 1 *14-ounce can coconut cream*
- ⅔ *cup coconut sugar or packed dark brown sugar*
- 2 *large eggs*
- ½ *teaspoon table salt*
- ½ *teaspoon ground cinnamon*
- ½ *teaspoon ground ginger*
- ¼ *teaspoon freshly grated nutmeg*
- ⅛ *teaspoon ground cloves*

Prepared pastry crust dough of your choice

1. Preheat the oven to 425°F.

2. Bring a large pot of water to a boil. Add the parsnips and cook until fork-tender, about 12–15 minutes. Drain the parsnips in a colander, then return to the pot and mash with a potato masher.

3. Measure out 2 cups of the parsnip mash and transfer to a food processor. (Reserve any remaining parsnips for another recipe or to add to a smoothie or pot of soup.) Add the coconut cream and process until smooth.

4. Pulse in the sugar, eggs, salt, cinnamon, ginger, nutmeg, and cloves, stopping when the mixture is smoothly combined.

5. Line a 9-inch tart pan with the prepared pastry crust. Using a fork, prick the bottom of the crust randomly. This will prevent bubbles by letting steam escape.

6. Bake the crust for 20 minutes.

7. Remove the tart pan from the oven, allow to cool for 10 minutes (you still want it to be a bit warm), then pour in the filling.

8. Lower the oven temperature to 350°F and bake the tart until the filling is almost set, about 45 minutes. You want the filling to be firm but still a bit jiggly. It will set as it cools; overcooking the tart will make for a tough, flavorless dessert.

9. Allow the tart to cool for at least an hour before cutting. This will help the flavors develop and firm up the texture. Serve with Whipped Coconut Topping (page 151), if desired.

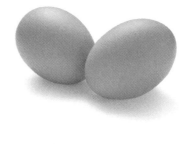

PURPLE SWEET POTATO PIE WITH COCONUT ALMOND CRUST

MAKES 8 SERVINGS

This is an outrageously dramatic pie, perhaps the most dramatic pie you will ever see. It calls for purple sweet potatoes, which give the dessert a bold violet color, but feel free to use regular orange sweet potatoes if that's what you have on hand.

Crust

1/4 cup liquid coconut oil

1/4 cup maple syrup, amber or dark

1 cup almond meal

1 cup unsweetened shredded coconut

1/2 teaspoon salt

1/2 teaspoon baking soda

Filling

2 pounds purple sweet potatoes, peeled and cut into 1-inch rounds (about 4 cups)

3/4 cup coconut cream

1/2 cup maple syrup, amber or dark

1 tablespoon tapioca starch

1 1/2 tablespoons fresh lemon juice

1/2 teaspoon salt

2 teaspoons ground cinnamon

1 teaspoon ground ginger

1/2 teaspoon allspice

1/4 teaspoon ground cloves

1. Preheat the oven to 350°F.

2. Very lightly grease the bottom and sides of a 9-inch pie pan with coconut oil.

3. Mix all the crust ingredients in a large bowl, then transfer them to the prepared pie pan. Wet your hands lightly to prevent the crust from sticking to them, then press the crust into the pan, making sure it is even on the sides and bottom.

4. Bake the crust for 10 minutes. When you remove it from the oven, the crust will have puffed up and be light golden brown. Use the back of a spoon to gently push the crust down so there is room for the filling.

5. Bring a medium-size pot of water to a boil. Add the sweet potatoes and boil for 10 minutes, or until they are easily pierced with a fork.

6. Remove the sweet potatoes and transfer to a food processor. Add the remaining filling ingredients and process until smooth. Taste the filling and adjust the sweetness (add a bit more syrup if you'd like) and spice.

7. Pour the pie filling into the baked pie shell and smooth out the top. Bake for 45 minutes, or until the pie has set but still has some jiggle in the middle. Remove the pie from the oven and let it cool completely before serving.

PUDDINGS

BAKED CINNAMON JICAMA

MAKES 4 SERVINGS

When sautéed and spiced with cinnamon, jicama can easily pass for apple. Here, it is spiced and served in dessert cups and dressed with a bit of Whipped Coconut Topping.

- 3 cups jicama, peeled and cubed
- ½ tablespoon lemon juice
- 3 tablespoons coconut oil
- ¼ cup coconut sugar
- 1 teaspoon pumpkin pie spice or apple pie spice

Whipped Coconut Topping (page 151)

1. Preheat the oven to 350°F.

2. In a large bowl, toss the jicama with the lemon juice, coconut oil, sugar, and spice.

3. Transfer the mixture to a small casserole or baking dish and bake, covered, for 25–30 minutes, or until just tender.

4. Serve with Whipped Coconut Topping.

BEET PANNA COTTA

MAKES 6 SERVINGS

This creamy dessert is a fun way to get beet-haters to eat their beets. If you want to change things up, feel free to use lemon or blood orange juice in place of the lime juice.

- 2 medium-size red beets (about ½ pound) trimmed and peeled
- ¼ teaspoon powdered ginger
- 2 cups coconut cream (one full can and part of a second)
- Pinch of salt
- 1 teaspoon unflavored gelatin
- 2 tablespoons cold water
- 3 tablespoons honey
- ½ teaspoon vanilla extract
- 1 tablespoon lime juice

Whipped Coconut Topping (optional), page 151

1. Roughly chop beets into half-inch pieces.

2. Add beets, ginger powder, coconut cream, and salt to a medium saucepan over medium-high heat. Bring to a simmer.

3. Cover, reduce heat to medium-low simmer and cook for about 25–30 minutes, or until beets are soft. Remove from heat and allow to cool 15 minutes.

4. While mixture is cooling, whisk together the gelatin and cold water in a small bowl. Let sit for 5 minutes to soften.

5. Add gelatin mixture, beet mixture, honey, vanilla, and lime juice to a blender. Puree until absolutely smooth.

6. Divide the puree evenly among 6 ramekins or dessert cups. Refrigerate for at least 4 hours.

7. If desired, serve with Whipped Coconut Topping.

CARROT CAKE PUDDING

MAKES 6 SERVINGS

This warm, spicy pudding is a bit like pumpkin pie in a cup, except it's made with carrots. This a tasty, health-supportive dessert that your entire family will love.

2   *teaspoons unflavored powdered gelatin*

1   *14-ounce can coconut cream*

¾   *cup packed shredded carrots*

½   *tablespoon vanilla extract*

¼   *cup honey*

2   *large egg yolks*

½   *teaspoon ground ginger*

¼   *teaspoon ground nutmeg*

¼   *teaspoon ground cinnamon*

Toasted coconut flakes (optional)

Toasted pecan pieces (optional)

Golden or Thompson raisins (optional)

1. Place 2 tablespoons of water in a bowl and sprinkle the gelatin on top. Set it aside to soften.

2. Combine the coconut cream and carrots in a medium saucepan over medium heat. Cook for 10 minutes, or until the carrots are soft.

3. Transfer the carrot mixture to a blender or food processor and process until smooth.

4. Whisk together the vanilla, honey, and egg yolks in a large bowl. Slowly whisk the carrot-coconut mixture into the egg mixture until both mixtures are completely combined.

5. Transfer the mixture to a saucepan over medium-low heat, stirring constantly and being careful not to let the mixture boil.

6. Stir in the ginger, nutmeg, cinnamon, and softened gelatin and whisk until completely dissolved. Cook for 5 minutes longer, or until the mixture is thick enough to coat a spoon or fork.

7. Transfer the mixture to a serving dish and place a layer of waxed paper or food wrap directly on the surface of the pudding. This will prevent a film from forming. Refrigerate for 6 hours to set.

8. Serve with coconut flakes, pecan pieces, and/or raisins.

CHOCOLATE-BEET-COCONUT PUDDING

MAKES 4 SERVINGS

This is the easiest way I know to get beets into kids. You'll need a juicer for this one—or you'll need to make a run to a juice joint that sells beet juice straight up.

- 2 cups chopped bittersweet chocolate or chocolate chips
- 1 cup coconut cream
- 1 teaspoon tapioca starch
- ½ teaspoon salt
- ½ cup red or orange beet juice (or a mix of the two)
- ½ teaspoon pure vanilla extract
- 1–2 tablespoons coconut sugar or cane sugar (optional)

1. Place the chocolate in a medium bowl. Set aside.

2. Add the coconut cream to a small saucepan over medium heat and cook for about 3 minutes, or until warm. Whisk in the tapioca starch and salt until dissolved. Continue cooking, stirring constantly, until the mixture thickens, about 2 minutes.

3. Stir in the beet juice and vanilla extract and whisk 1 minute more. Strain into the chocolate chips; let stand 1 minute, then whisk until the chocolate is smooth.

4. Taste, and add the sugar (if using) immediately while the mixture is warm. Whisk until dissolved.

5. Divide the pudding among four 6-ounce ramekins. Chill until cold.

SWEET POTATO INDIAN PUDDING

MAKES 6 SERVINGS

Indian pudding is a favorite traditional New England dessert made with cornmeal and molasses. It is homey and delicious. Here, it is made even yummier (and healthier) with sweet potato. I sometimes serve this as a brunch dish.

- 2 large sweet potatoes, baked until soft
- 2 14-ounce cans coconut milk
- ½ cup cornmeal
- 2 tablespoons coconut oil
- ¼ cup coconut sugar or maple syrup, amber or dark
- 2 tablespoons molasses or coconut nectar
- 1½ teaspoons cinnamon
- ½ teaspoon ground ginger
- ½ teaspoon nutmeg
- ½ teaspoon salt
- 3 eggs, room temperature
- ½ cup coconut cream

1. Preheat the oven to 275°F.

2. Remove the peel from the sweet potatoes and add to a food processor with the coconut milk. Process until smooth.

3. Transfer the sweet potato mixture to a large saucepan over medium heat. Whisk in the cornmeal, and bring to a boil, whisking constantly. Reduce the heat to medium-low and continue to whisk as you cook for 5–10 minutes, until thickened. Remove from the heat.

4. Add the coconut oil, maple syrup, molasses, cinnamon, ginger, nutmeg, and salt. Whisk until the mixture is completely blended. Remove from the heat.

5. In a separate small bowl, beat the eggs. Add about ½ cup of the warm cornmeal mixture to the eggs and beat again. Add the egg-cornmeal mixture back to the larger pot of cornmeal pudding and whisk together to combine.

6. Whisk in the coconut cream.

7. Grease the bottom of a large casserole dish. Scrape in the batter and smooth the top with a spatula. Bake for 2 hours. Serve warm, alone or with Whipped Coconut Topping (page 151).

FROZEN CONFECTIONS

JUICE POP BLUEPRINT

MAKES 6 SERVINGS

If you have a juicer, these will be a cinch. This is more of a blueprint than a recipe: You simply juice your favorite roots (beets and carrots do well in this recipe), mix with your choice of companion liquid, pour into ice pop molds, and wait for your yummy treat to be ready.

1½ cups unsweetened fruit juice

One envelope (2 teaspoons) unflavored gelatin

1   cup root juice

1. Warm the fruit juice in a small saucepan over medium heat. Once it is warm, remove from the heat and whisk in the gelatin, stirring until the gelatin dissolves.

2. Immediately whisk in the root juice.

3. Divide the mixture between six ice pop molds.

4. Place the molds in the freezer for 3 hours or more to harden.

NUTTY SWEET POTATO ICE CREAM

MAKES 4 SERVINGS

This yummy ice cream is very adaptable. You can use another root veggie or a different nut butter if you'd like.

- *½ cup cooked sweet potato, skin removed*
- *1 cup crunch or creamy no-additive peanut, almond, cashew, or sunflower butter*
- *½ cup maple syrup (or more as needed), amber or dark*
- *1 14-ounce can coconut cream*
- *1 tablespoon vanilla extract*
- *1 teaspoon cinnamon or pumpkin pie spice (optional)*
- *½ cup crushed nuts, coconut flakes, chopped chocolate, berries, and/or anything else that sounds yummy (optional)*

1. Combine the sweet potato, peanut butter, maple syrup, coconut cream, vanilla, and spice (if using) to a food processor and process until smooth. Taste for sweetness and add more sweetener if you so desire.

2. Transfer the mixture to an ice cream maker, add any optional add-ins, and freeze according to the manufacturer's instructions.

ROOT JUICE GELATO

MAKES ABOUT 3 CUPS

This is a fun, customizable recipe that uses nourishing coconut cream (or coconut milk, for a lighter version) with your favorite veggie juice (or juices). If you don't have a juicer, you can use juice bought at a juice joint.

- *1 14-ounce can coconut cream or coconut milk*
- *1–4 tablespoons sweetener of your choice*
- *4 teaspoons cornstarch or tapioca starch*
- *1½ cups root juice*
- *1 tablespoon lemon, lime, or orange juice*

1. Combine ¼ cup of the coconut cream, sweetener, and tapioca starch and whisk until smooth.

2. Add the remaining coconut cream to a small saucepan over low heat and cook just until small bubbles appear around the edge of the liquid.

3. Whisk the coconut cream–sweetener mixture into the coconut cream in the saucepan and allow to cook until the mixture thickens, about 5 minutes.

4. Once it appears to be thickening, remove it immediately from the heat and whisk in the root juice and lemon juice. Refrigerate until chilled.

5. Process in your ice cream machine according to the manufacturer's directions.

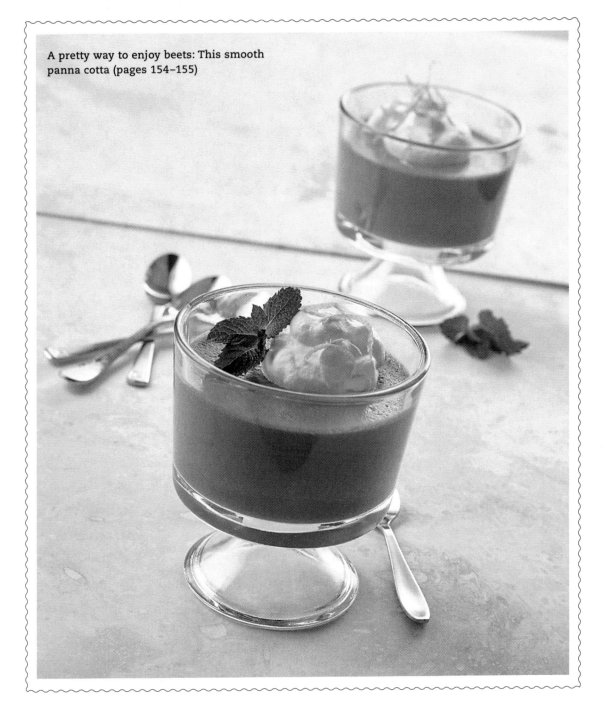

A pretty way to enjoy beets: This smooth
panna cotta (pages 154–155)

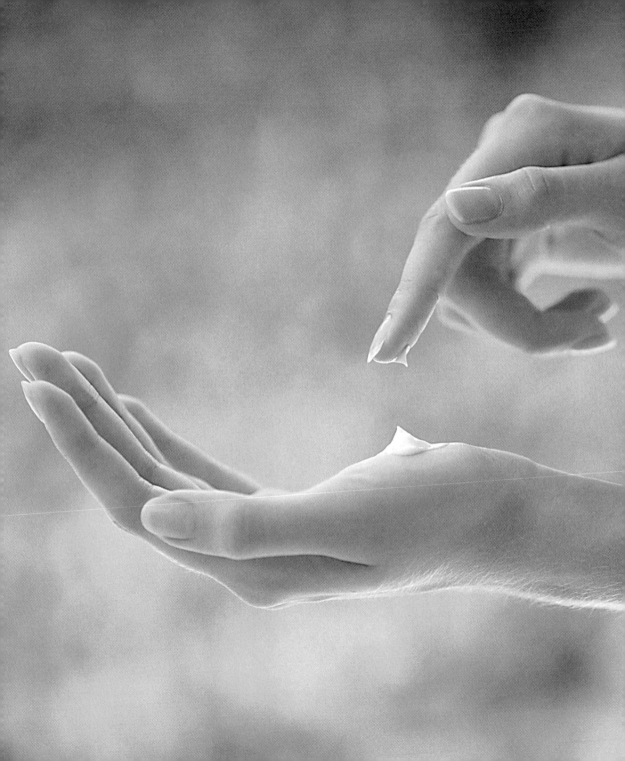

CHAPTER 9

BEAUTY

Root vegetables are high in antioxidants—nutrients that heal wounds, encourage healthy skin cell growth, repair collagen, lighten discoloration, and help maintain strong, vigorous hair growth. Sure, you could head to a health food store and buy a carrot-oil-infused moisturizer or a beet-based shower gel, but you'll have so much fun making your own. It's easy!

BODY CARE

ACNE-FIGHTING TAPIOCA BODY WASH

MAKES 1 CUP

Tapioca—cassava root that has been dried and pulverized—absorbs oil and waste material, making it fantastic for cleaning up clogged pores and clearing acne. This easy recipe uses liquid castile soap, but if you'd like, you can simply add the tapioca starch to your favorite bath gel.

8 ounces liquid castile soap

2 tablespoons tapioca starch

5 drops of your favorite essential oil (optional)

1. Whisk all ingredients together in a mixing bowl.

2. Transfer to a squeeze bottle and keep in your bathroom.

3. There is no need to refrigerate, but shake the bottle before using.

NOTE: When using food-based beauty treatments, be sure to collect any solid material and discard it properly (preferably in a compost bin!). Rolled oats, grated jicama, and the like can really clog up sinks and shower drains!

OPPOSITE: **Before using any self-care item, it is helpful to test it on your skin first, then wait an hour to see if you develop a reaction**

BURDOCK BATH SOAK

MAKES ENOUGH FOR ONE BATH

Burdock is a wonderful detoxifying plant. When used on the body, it can help draw impurities and trapped matter out of the pores so skin can heal.

1 *burdock root, scrubbed clean and roughly chopped*

1. Place the burdock root in a small saucepan over medium-high heat and add 3 cups of water.

2. Bring to a boil.

3. Cover the pot and turn off the heat. Allow the pot to sit undisturbed for 2–3 hours while the burdock steeps.

4. Remove the burdock pieces (for a quick facial mask, you can puree them and stir in enough honey to form a paste).

5. Fill the bathtub with warm water. Add the burdock liquid directly to bath.

CARROT OIL

MAKES ABOUT ¼ CUP

Carrot oil is a well-known beauty aid that is high in carotenes and antioxidants. It is great for adding moisture to skin and calming irritated or sunburned skin. (According to folk remedies, massaging carrot oil into your scalp can even stimulate hair growth!) Note that you'll need a few supplies for this recipe.

2 *large carrots, trimmed and peeled*
Extra virgin olive oil

1. Place the carrots in a food processor and pulse until coarsely ground, or use the food processor's grater attachment and grate them.

2. Place the grated carrots in a slow cooker and pour in just enough oil to cover the carrots (this is usually more than 2 cups).

3. Place your slow cooker on its lowest setting, which for most slow cookers is "warm." Set the timer, if your slow cooker has one, for 24 hours. During this time, the oil will be infused with the carrots' nutrients.

4. Line a fine-mesh strainer with cheesecloth and set it over a clean bowl. Using a silicone spatula, scrape the carrots and oil into the strainer and let the oil drip into the bowl. If you need to, take the cheesecloth out of the strainer and squeeze any extra carrot oil into the bowl.

5. Scrape the oil into a clean glass jar or pot. Store in the refrigerator for up to 6 months.

6. Use on rough patches, rashes, under your eyes, around your cuticles, or wherever else you'd like.

FACIAL CARE

CARROT MASK

MAKES ONE APPLICATION

This brightly colored mask is a lovely way to brighten skin, lighten discoloration, and ward off breakouts.

1 carrot, trimmed

1 tablespoon honey

Juice of ½ lemon

1. Roughly chop the carrot and either place in a steamer basket and cook until soft, or boil in a very small amount of water until soft.

2. Scrape the cooked carrots and any liquid into the bowl of a food processor or blender. Add the honey and lemon juice and process until smooth.

3. Apply immediately to clean, dry skin.

4. Allow the mask to remain on for 20 minutes. Remove with a warm, wet washcloth.

OATMEAL-BEET EXFOLIATING MASK

MAKES ONE APPLICATION

I feel the need to warn you how messy this mask is. But, the results are worth the fuchsia mess it makes: You'll have bright, tight, moist, glowing skin.

½ cup fresh-grated beet (or use fresh pulp from the juicer)

½ cup rolled oats

1½ teaspoons coconut milk, coconut water, or plain water

1. Mix all ingredients together in a bowl until combined.

2. Apply immediately to clean, dry skin. With wet fingers, massage the mask into the skin.

3. Allow the mask to remain on for 20 minutes. You may need to recline in order to keep the mask from sliding off your face onto your clothing, the furniture, and the floor.

4. Remove the mask with a warm, wet washcloth. Splash your face with warm water if necessary to remove bits of oatmeal and beet root.

JICAMA BRIGHTENER

MAKES ONE APPLICATION

Jicama is a traditional folk remedy for bright, firm, youthful skin and is used in many cultures to lighten discoloration.

½ small jicama, freshly grated

1. Apply immediately to clean, dry skin.

2. Allow the mask to remain on for 20 minutes. You may need to recline in order to keep the mask from sliding off your face onto your clothing, the furniture, and the floor.

3. Remove with a warm, wet washcloth.

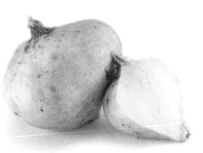

HAIR CARE

HAIR DETOXIFIER

MAKES ONE APPLICATION

Once in a while, your normally well-behaved hair may look dry and scraggly. Frizzy. Unruly. Not shiny. You haven't done anything different, but still, your hair doesn't look as good as it usually does. This treatment can help. It's kind of weird and it's definitely messy (use a drain catcher!), but it does restore hair's liveliness. You'll need a shower cap for this one.

1 large carrot, trimmed and grated

1. Start with clean (or "pretty clean") hair. Rub the grated carrot onto your scalp, making sure to get the areas above your ears and behind them. Rub the remaining carrot down the length of your hair and tuck your hair into a shower cap. If you do not have a shower cap, tie your hair in a bandana.

2. Wait about 20 minutes or more. Rinse your hair in the shower using cool water. No need to shampoo.

ROOTY DRY SHAMPOO

MAKES ABOUT 10 APPLICATIONS

We use a lot of dry shampoo in our house. Before you judge, let me say that yes, we do wash our hair. But I've got teens whose hair always looks oily to me. Instead of spending money on chemical-laden spray-on dry shampoo or using baby powder (talc has been linked to cancer), we use homemade dry shampoo, based on dried cassava root (also known as tapioca). This works best on light brown, blond, and gray hair. If you have dark hair, add a few teaspoons of cocoa powder to the mix. This will ensure your hair doesn't take on a gray cast from the dry shampoo.

½ cup tapioca starch

5–6 drops of your favorite essential oil (optional)

2–3 teaspoons cocoa (optional, for dark hair)

1. Add the tapioca starch to a clean, sealable glass container.

2. If using essential oil and/or cocoa powder, add that to the jar. Gently shake to blend.

3. To use, sprinkle 1–2 teaspoons around the roots of your hair and massage into your scalp. Bend over and give your head a good shake to get rid of any excess powder.

4. Repeat in other areas as needed.

5. Store tightly sealed in a dry place.

SHINE AND BODY RINSE

MAKES ONE APPLICATION

This easy rinse creates a lot of shine—especially on gray hair. It also bulks up the hair, creating body, making it a good solution for finer strands. One of the best things about it is how easy it is: Next time you're cooking potatoes for dinner, simply save the cooking water!

1 pound or more potatoes, any color, cut in half or quarters

1. Place the potatoes in a large pot and fill with water to cover.

2. Place the pot over medium-high heat and boil the potatoes until they are fork-tender.

3. Using a slotted spoon, remove the potatoes and reserve them for another use. I am sure you can find a recipe in this book to use them in!

4. Allow the liquid to cool. Place the pot in the refrigerator if you'd like.

5. Transfer the cooled liquid to a shatterproof bottle and take it into the shower with you.

6. Wash and condition your hair as usual, then finish up by dousing your hair with the entire amount of potato liquid, making sure to soak all strands. No need to rinse out.

7. Dry and style your hair as usual.

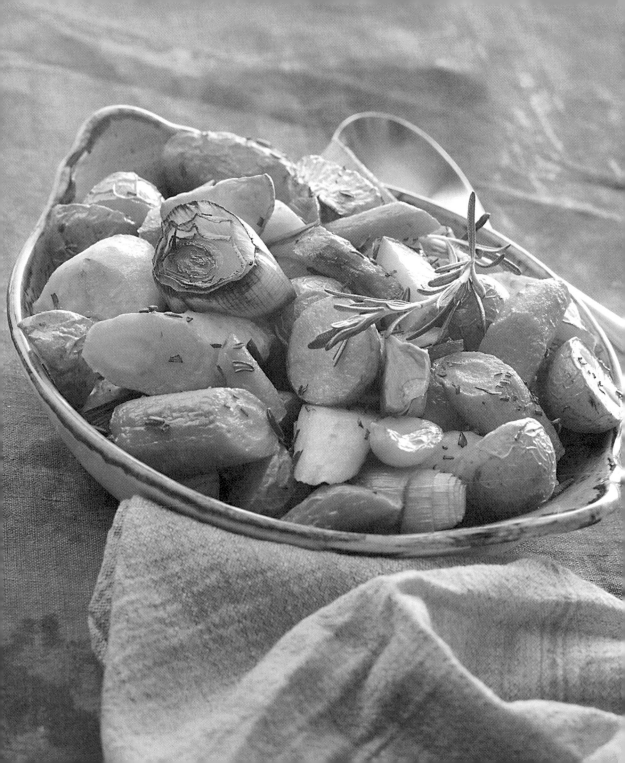

CHAPTER 10

FREQUENTLY ASKED QUESTIONS

Humans have been eating roots of all kinds since the beginning of time. That doesn't mean we know everything about them, though. Here are some of the most common questions I am asked about root vegetables.

What is the difference between a root and a bulb?

A vegetable root grows underground and anchors the plant and all of its parts that grow above it. The plant absorbs nutrients and moisture from the soil around it.

A bulb, as one of my kids' science teachers explained it, is next year's plant safely packaged and surrounded by white fleshy scales that contain all the food that the bulb needs. Deeper into the interior of the bulb are immature leaves, flower stems, and sometimes even flower buds. At the base of the bulb is a flat section, often with a few visible hairy tentacle-like roots, called a basal plate. This is the bulb's root. Think of an onion or fennel bulb: When you cut these in half lengthwise, you can see all of these inside. Bulbs can grow under the ground or at ground level.

What is the difference between a root and a rhizome?

As stated above, a root is an organ of the plant—usually found underground—that has no leaves or nodes. A rhizome is made up of the same tissues as a stem and typically grows horizontally under the earth or at ground level. Popular culinary rhizomes include ginger root (a misnomer, since it's not really a root), fresh turmeric, and galangal.

Can all roots be eaten?

No. There are about 50 types of storage roots commonly eaten around the world and a handful of others that, while not particularly tasty, can be consumed in a pinch. But there are many more roots (more than we have space for in this book) that, while plump and edible-looking, cause reactions that range from mild diarrhea and cramps to anaphylactic shock and a slowing or stopping of the heart. If eating wild edible roots appeals to you, get some training and go out with someone who has experience in this realm. If you're not sure about something, don't put it in your mouth!

Can all edible roots be enjoyed raw?

No. Many of the roots in this book are wonderful both cooked and raw, including beets, burdock, celeriac, parsnips, salsify, turnip, and more. But there are a number of edible roots that must to be cooked before they are enjoyed. Cassava—featured in this book—is one of them. Known also as manioc or yuca (not the similar-sounding yucca, which is an entirely different plant, one that grows throughout the western United States deserts), it contains traces of a cyanide-like plant chemical that is deactivated in the presence of heat. Thus cassava is always boiled, baked, fried, roasted, or sautéed. I have noted throughout the book which roots can be enjoyed raw and which should be cooked. I want you to be both healthy and safe!

Can the leaves of root vegetables be eaten?

Not all of them are edible. Many taste just plain bad. Others can cause severe gastric distress, skin reactions, or worse. Throughout the book I've noted which leaves are good to eat—you'll even find recipes for them—and which are not, but here's a quick list.

ENJOY

Beet greens: Enjoy cooked.

Burdock greens (only young leaves; the mature leaves are so bitter they can cause stomach upset): Cook or use as a salad green.

Carrot tops: Lovely juiced or minced into sauces or salads.

Celeriac tops: Use anywhere you'd use regular celery.

Radish leaves: The peppery flavor reminds me of arugula. Sauté, juice, or use in salads.

Rutabaga: Good as a pot green.

Salsify and Scorzonera: The young, tender leaves are nice in salads.

Sweet potato leaves: A mild sautéed green.

Turnip greens: Wonderful as a pot green.

IGNORE

Cassava greens: Cassava greens contain high amounts of a chemical related to cyanide. Handling them can cause a skin reaction. While the root is safe to eat cooked, the leaves are not.

Parsnip greens: Handling parsnip greens and stems can cause a very strong phototoxic reaction, thanks to a substance found in the aboveground part of the plant. It is best not to even touch this part of the plant without wearing gloves. As for eating, there are mixed opinions on whether it is safe. Err on the side of caution and find another green to enjoy.

Potato tops: The aboveground part of the potato plant contains large amounts of a substance called solanine, an alkaloid that can cause gastric distress, headache, shock, and even paralysis.

I like to gather wild foods. How do I know if a root is poisonous?

Often there is no reliable way to tell. If wild-gathering is something you enjoy, go with a trusted expert who has a proven track record.

What is the most widely eaten root vegetable in the world?

If production is any indicator of consumption, it may be the potato. According to the Food and Agriculture Organization of the United Nations (FAO), 385 million metric tons were grown commercially around the world in 2014 (with similar amounts grown in earlier years). This includes not only the superfood varieties featured in this book (purple, gold, and red-flesh), but the traditional russet potato, as well.

Runners-up go to carrots and turnips. The FAO reports that 36 million metric tons were grown commercially.

I do a lot of gardening. Is there a way of keeping ground-dwelling animals from eating my root vegetables?

Voles, moles, shrews, and mice are some of the most common reasons you have no root veggies to harvest. It's important to remember that you cannot garden without running into evidence of one or more of these varmints. Just knowing that does help.

A multipronged strategy works best:

• Many of these animals need ground cover, so remove as much of it as pssible.

• Get two cats, who will help scare off many of these, especially if the cats are allowed to stay in the garden at night, when a lot of these pests are active.

• Get a dog, who can help guard the garden against deer.

• Sonic spikes (look for solar-powered versions) emit frequencies below the ground that keep away rodents.

• Use raised beds.

• Fence in your garden with ¼-inch mesh fencing. Your fence should be at least 1 foot high aboveground. Drive fence stakes at least 6 inches into the ground and bend the fencing inward belowground into an L shape.

My garden has produced more root veggies than I can use. Can I freeze them for later? How do I do that?

Absolutely! Potatoes don't freeze well—they get both grainy and mushy—but all other root veggies freeze beautifully. Start by putting a very large pot of salted water on the stove over high heat. While you are waiting for the water to come to a vigorous, rolling boil, place a large colander in the sink under the faucet.

Next, turn your attention to your roots. Start by cleaning the vegetables and trimming away their greens and any unappetizing spots or sprouts. Peel (or not) and cut into the size you'd like. When the water is boiling, plunge 1–2 cups of roots into the boiling water (use a blanching basket if you'd like, or grab a spider or slotted spoon to fish out veggies). The water will probably stop boiling. Wait until it starts simmering again and count to 60. Quickly remove the veggies and place in the waiting colander. Turn on the cold water and shower the veggies until they are cool to the touch, shaking the colander a few times so the veggies on the bottom are washed in cold water, too. Allow to dry and place directly in a freezer storage container or bag. Use within 6 months.

Why are root vegetables considered superfoods? Is it because they contain fiber, vitamins, and minerals?

The fiber, vitamins, and minerals in root vegetables (of all kinds) make them a very healthy food. However, what make them superfoods are plant chemicals called phytonutrients, powerful antioxidants that help strengthen the immune system, prevent cardiovascular conditions, create a strong nervous system, protect against cancer, heal the skin and eyes, and so much more.

Can you talk a bit more about phytonutrients?

Plant foods contain vitamins and minerals that are essential to keeping humans alive. Plants also contain something that—while not essential to human life—helps prevent disease and keeps our bodies working properly. These are plant chemicals called phytonutrients, or phytochemicals. They help protect plants from bacteria, viruses, germs, fungi, bugs, drought, and temperature fluctuations. It is believed that more than 25,000 phytonutrients are found in plant foods. Six of the most important kinds of phytonutrients include carotenoids, ellagic acid, flavonoids, resveratrol, glucosinolates, and phytoestrogens.

Can eating too many roots be harmful to my health?

Well, eating too much of anything can be, but even so, it's unlikely. Even avid veggie eaters would be hard-pressed to eat large enough quantities to cause problems. Individuals with diabetes and other blood sugar conditions will probably want to limit their consumption of the sweeter roots—beets and carrots—to no more than two servings daily, and eating more than five or six servings of carrots or sweet potatoes daily can induce a condition called carotenia, a temporarily orange tinge of the skin due to the beta-carotene in the veggies. Before increasing your root consumption, however, be safe and speak with your healthcare provider.

I have a stove that measures temperatures in Celsius. Do you have a metric conversion chart I can refer to?

Fahrenheit	Celsius
200°	100°
225°	110°
250°	130°
275°	140°
300°	150°
325°	160°
350°	180°
375°	190°
400°	200°
425°	220°
450°	250°

PHOTO CREDITS

www.agmrc.org

The Agricultural Marketing Resource Center features everything you could want to know about agricultural food production in the United States, from growing to using to marketing efforts.

www.ams.usda.gov/local-food-directories/farmersmarkets

The National Farmers Market Directory makes it easy to find a nearby source for your favorite root vegetables.

www.carrotmuseum.co.uk

This online "museum" features everything you ever wanted to know about carrots, from growing info to recipes to history.

www.catefarm.com/burdock-and-echinacea

Cate Farm, in East Montpelier, Vermont, is one of the few farms in the United States that specializes in burdock.

www.garden.org

At the National Gardening Association's website you can learn about all the root veggies, as well as all kinds of other plants.

www.growingtaste.com

A fantastic site for the home gardener. Learn how to choose, grow, harvest, store, and enjoy your favorite root (and other) veggies, including celeriac, sweet potato, scorzonera, salsify, and sunchoke.

www.harvesttotable.com

Harvest to Table is aimed at helping home gardeners grow and enjoy their own food. They've got great information on root vegetables, including facts about the more esoteric roots, such as salsify and sunchoke.

www.hvfarmhub.org/extending-the-growing-season-through-root-crops

Located in New York State, Hudson Valley Farm Hub is an organization dedicated to bringing education to farmers and gardeners.

www.nationalpotatocouncil.org

The National Potato Council's site features information for both growers and consumers. Learn about the different type of potatoes, as well as potato resources such as festivals, publications, and more.

www.stephaniepedersen.com

This is the author's own site, which includes information on her books and her nutrition practice, as well as plenty of superfood recipes.

www.whfoods.com

World's Healthiest Foods is a megasite of nutrition stats, studies, and discussions about superfoods.

METRIC CONVERSION CHARTS

METRIC EQUIVALENTS—LIQUID

U.S. QUANTITY	METRIC EQUIVALENT	U.S. QUANTITY	METRIC EQUIVALENT
¼ teaspoon	1 ml	¼ cup	60 ml
½ teaspoon	2.5 ml	⅓ cup	80 ml
¾ teaspoon	4 ml	½ cup	120 ml
1 teaspoon	5 ml	⅔ cup	160 ml
1¼ teaspoons	6 ml	¾ cup	180 ml
1½ teaspoons	7.5 ml	1 cup	240 ml
1¾ teaspoons	8.5 ml	1½ cups	350 ml
2 teaspoons	10 ml	3 cups	700 ml
1 tablespoon	15 ml	4 cups	950 ml
2 tablespoons	30 ml		

METRIC EQUIVALENTS—DRY

INGREDIENT	¼ CUP	⅓ CUP	½ CUP	⅔ CUP	¾ CUP	1 CUP
GRAINS AND GRAIN PRODUCTS (UNCOOKED)						
All-purpose flour	31 g	42 g	62 g	83 g	94 g	125 g
Millet	50 g	67 g	100 g	133 g	150 g	200 g
Oats, rolled	25 g	33 g	50 g	67 g	75 g	100 g
Quinoa	42 g	57 g	85 g	113 g	127 g	170 g
Rice: brown, black, red	48 g	63 g	95 g	127 g	142 g	190 g
NUTS AND SEEDS						
Almonds, chopped	35 g	47 g	70 g	93 g	105 g	140 g
Pepitas (hulled pumpkin seeds, whole	35 g	46 g	69 g	92 g	104 g	138 g
Sunflower seeds, hulled, whole	32 g	43 g	64 g	85 g	96 g	128 g
Walnuts, chopped	31 g	42 g	62 g	83 g	94 g	125 g
SWEETENERS						
Brown sugar, firmly packed	55 g	73 g	110 g	147 g	165 g	220 g
Coconut sugar	50 g	67 g	100 g	133 g	150 g	200 g
Granulated sugar	50 g	67 g	100 g	133 g	150 g	200 g

ACKNOWLEDGMENTS

I couldn't have finished *Roots: The Complete Guide to the Underground Superfood* without the support of many special people. First, a shout-out to my husband, Richard Joseph Demler, and our sons Leif Christian Pedersen, Anders Gyldenvalde Pedersen, and Axel SuneLund Pedersen. Richard, you are amazing. When it became clear that I was struggling to finish this book in a timely manner, you took our beautiful (but not always well-behaved) boys down to Virginia for three entire weeks, which allowed me to write, cook, and edit without interruption. I am incredibly grateful to you for everything.

Thanks to so many friends who supported my family and me during the book-writing process. Oceana, our morning check-ins are so powerful. They allow me to sit down to a day of writing with a sense of focus and fun. C. Baker . . . Thank you! Thank you! Thank you! For everything.

Thanks to my amazing clients for the constant inspiration you bring. I am in awe of each of you!

I can't say enough flattering (and true!) things about my gorgeous, good-humored, brilliant editor, Hannah Reich, who is also a fellow healthy food lover. Also, thanks to Sterling's Jennifer Williams. We go back in time through several publishing houses now. I count my blessings that I was assigned, as a young author, to you all those years ago. Here's to us! My designers Christine Heun and Wendy Ralphs ensured that this book was as polished and professional as possible. Photographer Bill Milne, with the help of food stylist Diane Vezza, turned my tasty recipes into the gorgeous, mouthwatering photos in *Roots: The Complete Guide to the Underground Superfood*. And my very thorough copy editor, Lori Paximadis, ensured that the book you hold in your hands is as good as possible. Thank you, everyone! Your calm, can-do demeanors and overall smarty-pants ways make this crazy business of publishing look glamorous.

Thanks so much to my publicity pro, Sherri McLendon, of Professional Moneta. Sherri, I adore our conversations. Not only are you fun and witty (and you know how much I love witty people), you make my professional life so much easier. Which in turn makes my profession al life more fun!

Lastly, I must thank you, dear reader and root lover, for your interest. Thank you!

—*Stephanie*

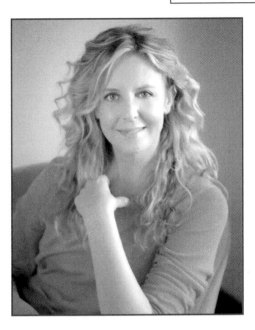

Stephanie Pedersen is a holistic nutritionist, food educator, cookbook author, corporate speaker, and media host. The author of more than twenty-two books, Stephanie has a reputation for teaching people how to make nutrition easy, practical, and fun. She does this by using superfoods and other "power foods" to help individuals detoxify naturally, manage food allergies, eliminate cravings, and lose weight using food and lifestyle changes.

According to Stephanie, getting healthy doesn't have to be complicated or time-consuming. "As a mother, writer, nutritionist, educator, and someone who loves to have time alone to wander local famers' markets, I know that complicated, overly fussy diets and an unnatural obsession with calorie-counting are not the answers to getting and staying healthy." Instead, Stephanie espouses a life of love, laughter, daily exercise, and your favorite whole foods (including plenty of superfoods!).

"We're lucky that we live at a time when more and more gorgeous whole food ingredients, organic products, and humanely farmed meats are available. Let's celebrate our good fortune by exploring our many food and fitness options and experimenting with abandon."

Pedersen currently lives in New York City with her husband and three sons. Visit her at www.StephaniePedersen.com for free gifts and classes, as well as to learn more about using foods and lifestyle actions to make your life healthier and happier. You can also learn more by tuning in to one of Stephanie's weekly radio shows—*Your Big Life* and *The Superfood Moment*—or stop by YouTube for her family health series, *Real Eating*, starring Stephanie and her sons.

Also by Stephanie Pedersen:

Berries: The Complete Guide to Cooking with Power-Packed Berries

The 7-Day Superfood Cleanse

Coconut: The Complete Guide to the World's Most Versatile Superfood

Kale: The Complete Guide to the World's Most Powerful Superfood

The Pumpkin Pie Spice Cookbook

NOTE: Page numbers in *italics* indicate photos separate from recipe. Page numbers in **bold** indicate nutrient characteristic summaries.

Acne-fighting body wash, 161
Alpha-carotene, **5**, 10, 35
Arrowroot, 18, 105, 140
Arthritis. *See* Inflammation, reducing
Athletic performance, improving, 2

Bacon. *See* Pork
Barley Bake, 131
Barley-Root Soup, 127
Beans and other legumes. *See also* Chickpeas
Beet Bean Burgers, 78
Beet-Bean Chili, 93–94
Cannellini Beet Dip, 117
Cannellini Veggie Sandwich, 84
Celeriac Lentil Salad, 123–124
Collard Root Wrap, 83
Easy Root Soup Blueprint, 95–96
Roasted Sweet Potato Salad with Chipotle Vinaigrette, 90–91
Root Veggie Pita, 84
Salmon on a Bed of Rooty Lentils, 142
Southwestern Salad, 125–126
Spiced Root Dal Soup, 130
Spicy Fish Taco Bowls, 88
Sweet Potato and Black Bean Breakfast Wraps, 65
Vegan Shepherd's Pie, 142–143
Beauty recipes, 161–165
Acne-Fighting Tapioca Body Wash, 161
Burdock Bath Soak, 162
Carrot Mask, 163
Hair Detoxifier, 164
Jicama Brightener, 164
Oatmeal-Beet Exfoliating mask, 163
Rooty Dry Shampoo, 165
Shine and Body Rinse, 165
Beef
Beef-and-Root Stew, 128
Beef-Root Burgers, 77–78
Braised Brisket and Roots, 140–141

Beets, 2–3
about: botanical background, 3; buying, 3; cooking oatmeal in juice of, 73; general information, 3; greens and their uses, 44, 168; growing information, 3; health-supporting role, 2–3; nutrition profile, 2; storing, 3; things to be aware of, 3; using/uses, x, 3, 44
Baked Root Chips, *98*, 102–103
Beef-Root Burgers, 77–78
Beet-and-Celeriac-Greens Smoothie, 43
Beet Bean Burgers, 78
Beet-Bean Chili, 93–94
Beet Cake, 145–146
Beet Chutney, 112
Beet-Date Ketchup, 115
Beet No-Wheat Scones, 51–52
Beet Panna Cotta, 154–155, *159*
Beetroot Latte, 41
Brunch Salad, 67
Cannellini Beet Dip, 117
Carrot Cake Muffins, *50*, 52
Chocolate-Beet-Coconut Pudding, 156
Collard Root Wrap, 83
Grain-Free Porridge, 73
Hearty Carrot Juice Pulp Crackers, 104
Oatmeal-Beet Exfoliating mask, 163
Red Smoothie, *40*, 46
Roasted Beet Waffles, 59
Rooty Buddha Bowl, 89
Rooty Pinwheels, 101
Salmon and Roasted Root Veggie Salad, 91–92
Shredded Root Salad Blueprint, 92–93
Southwestern Salad, 125–126
Sweet Root Chia Pudding, 75
Veggie Thin Crackers, 105
Warm Root Salad, 70
Berries, in GORP Carrot Chips, 99
Berries, in Red Smoothie, *40*, 46
Beta-carotene, 2, **5**, 10, 12, 17, 22, 25, 28, 33, 35
Blood pressure, 2, 3, 6, 7, 23, 25
Body care. *See* Beauty recipes

Bone health, 15. *See also* Calcium; Fluoride; Manganese; Phosphorus; Vitamin K
Bowel movements, regularity, 36
Bowls, 86–89
Breakfast, 51–75
about: types/forms of oats, 74
Autumn Spice Oatmeal, 71
Beet No-Wheat Scones, 51–52
Breakfast Quinoa, 71–72
Breakfast Tapioca, 72
Brunch Salad, 67
Cabbage-Carrot Frittata with Rosemary, 61
Carrot Cake Muffins, *50*, 52
Carrot Cake Oatmeal, 72–73
Carrot Cake Waffles, 56
Celeriac Hash, 62
Classy Hash, 63
Glory Muffins, 53
Grain-Free Porridge, 73
Mexicali Rutabaga Muffins, 54
Parsnip Griddle Cakes, 57
Parsnip Salmon Pancakes, 58
Roasted Beet Waffles, 59
Roasted Root Vegetables with Ham, 64
Rooty Breakfast Cake, 55
Rooty Rolled Oat Risotto, 67–68
Sweet Potato and Black Bean Breakfast Wraps, 65
Sweet Potato Hash with Eggs, 66
Sweet Root Chia Pudding, 75
Turnip Latkes, 60
Warm Root Salad, 70
Bulbs confused with roots, 32, 167
Burdock, 8–10
about: botanical background, 10; buying, 9; general information, 9–10; greens and their uses, 44; growing information, 10; health-supporting role, 8–9; history of, 10; nutrition profile, 8; storing, 9; things to be aware of, 10; using/uses, x, 9, 10, 44; Velcro origin and, 95
Barley Bake, 131
Braised Brisket and Roots, 140–141

Burdock Bath Soak, 162
Burdock or Salsify Relish, 110–111
Burdock Tea, 42
Carrot-Burdock Bisque, 94–95
Homemade Burdock and Dandelion Soda, 42
Rooty Buddha Bowl, 89
Burgers. *See* Sandwiches and wraps

Cabbage-Carrot Frittata with Rosemary, 61
Calcium, **5**, 15, 28, 30, 35
Cancer
breast, 9, 15, 37–38
colon, 17, 28
fighting/killing cells, 15, 17, 36, 37
leukemia, 20, 36
lung, 38
preventing/reducing risk, 4, 5, 6, 9, 10–11, 13, 15, 17, 28, 31, 36, 37–38
prostate, 10–11, 38
shrinking tumors, 13, 28
Candida, 34
Caponata, 114
Carrots, 10–12
about: botanical background, 11; breakfast side dishes, 69; buying, 11; cooking oatmeal in juice of, 73; general information, 11–12; greens and their uses, 44, 113, 168; growing information, 12; health-supporting role, 10–11; history of, 12; nutrition profile, 10; plate of sticks, 69; storing, 11; things to be aware of, 12; using/uses, 11, 12, 44, 113
Barley-Root Soup, 127
Beef-and-Root Stew, 128
Beef-Root Burgers, 77–78
Beetroot Latte, 41
Braised Brisket and Roots, 140–141
Cabbage-Carrot Frittata with Rosemary, 61
Cannellini Veggie Sandwich, 84
Carrot-Burdock Bisque, 94–95
Carrot Cake Muffins, *50*, 52

Carrot Cake Oatmeal, 72–73
Carrot Cake Pudding, 155
Carrot Cake Waffles, 56
Carrot Falafel Balls, 79
Carrot-Hazelnut Puree, 135
Carrot-Mango Lassi, *40*, 45
Carrot Mask, 163
Carrot-Orange Juice, 49
Carrot Pie, 151
Carrot Spread, 118
Classy Hash, 63
Collard Root Wrap, 83
Fresh Green Sauce, 113
GORP Carrot Chips, 99
Grain-Free Porridge, 73
Grated Carrot Salad, 69
Hair Detoxifier, 164
Healthier Carrot Cake, *144*,
    148
Hearty Carrot Juice Pulp
    Crackers, 104
Mexican Pickled Carrots and
    Jalapeños, *106*, 107
Moroccan Quinoa with
    Roots, 133
Parsnip-Carrot Pickle, 108
Roast Chicken and Root
    Vegetables with Mustard-
    Rosemary Sauce, 139
Roasted Root Vegetables, 136
Roasted Root Vegetables
    with Ham, 64
Root Veggie Pita, 84
Rooty Breakfast Cake, 55
Rooty Buddha Bowl, 89
Rooty Pinwheels, 101
Salmon on a Bed of Rooty
    Lentils, 142
Shredded Root Salad
    Blueprint, 92–93
Southwestern Salad, 125–126
Spiced Root Dal Soup, 130
Sweet Root Chia Pudding,
    75
Turkish Celeriac, 138
Vegan Shepherd's Pie,
    142–143
Veggie Fusion Juice, 49
Veggie Thin Crackers, 105
Warm Root Salad, 70
Cassava, 12–14
    about: botanical background,
    14; buying, 13; general
    information, 13–14;
    greens precaution, 44, 168;
    growing information, 14;
    health-supporting role,
    12–13; nutrition profile,
    12; storing, 13; things to be

aware of, 14; using/uses, 14,
    44; worldwide, 14
Acne-Fighting Tapioca Body
    Wash, 161
Breakfast Tapioca, 72
Rooty Dry Shampoo, 165
Cauliflower, 129
Celeriac, 15–16
    about: botanical background,
    16; buying, 15–16; general
    information, 15–16; greens
    and their uses, 44; health-
    supporting role, 15; history
    of, 16; nutrition profile, 15;
    storing, 16; things to be
    aware of, 16; using/uses,
    16, 44, 62
Autumn Quinoa Bowl, 87
Baked Root Chips, *98*,
    102–103
Barley-Root Soup, 127
Beet-and-Celeriac-Greens
    Smoothie, 43
Celeriac Hash, 62
Celeriac Juice, 48
Celeriac Lentil Salad,
    123–124
Celeriac Salad, 69
Hearty Carrot Juice Pulp
    Crackers, 104
Roasted Root Vegetables, 136
Roasted Root Vegetables with
    Ham, 64
Root Veggie Pita, 84
Rooty Pinwheels, 101
Sauté of Root Vegetables, 137
Turkish Celeriac, 138
Vegan Shepherd's Pie,
    142–143
Veggie Thin Crackers, 105
Warm Root Salad, 70
Chicken, roast with root
    vegetables, 139
Chickpeas
    about: hummus uses, 121
    Carrot Falafel Balls, 79
    Root Vegetable Curry, 141
    Root Veggie Pita, 84
    Rooty Buddha Bowl, 89
    Shredded Root Salad
    Blueprint, 92–93
    Sweet Potato Hummus,
    120–121
    Sweet Potato Protein Burgers,
    76, 82
Chili. *See* Soups, stews, and
    chilis
Chocolate-Beet-Coconut
    Pudding, 156

Cholesterol, 5, 6, 7, 8
Choline, 2, **5**, 8, 10, 12, 15, 17,
    20, 22, 25, 28, 33, 35, 37
Citrus
    Carrot-Orange Juice, 49
    PPL Juice, 48
    Radish Jicama Juice, 47
    Red Smoothie, *40*, 46
    Rutabaga Juice Cocktail, 47
Coconut
    about: coconut sugar tips, 146
    Chocolate-Beet-Coconut
    Pudding, 156
    Coconut Cream Frosting,
    150
    Purple Sweet Potato Pie with
    Coconut Almond Crust,
    153
    Whipped Coconut Topping,
    151
Coffee, in Beetroot Latte, 41
Cognitive decline, stopping, 15
Collard Root Wrap, 83
Condiments and sauces,
    107–121
    about: hummus uses, 121;
    make-ahead veggie dippers
    and, 114
    Beet Chutney, 112
    Beet-Date Ketchup, 115
    Burdock or Salsify Relish,
    110–111
    Cannellini Beet Dip, 117
    Carrot Spread, 118
    Chipotle Vinaigrette, 90–91
    Creamy Cream-Free Radish
    Dip, 118
    Fresh Green Sauce, 113
    Mexican Pickled Carrots and
    Jalapeños, *106*, 107
    Parsnip-Carrot Pickle, 108
    Pesto, 63
    Pickled Turnips, 109
    Radish-Jicama Salsa, 112
    Sunchoke Pickles, 109–110
    Superfood Caponata, 114
    Superfood Skordalia, 119
    Sweet Potato Hummus,
    120–121
    Sweet Potato Mustard, 116
Constipations, 36
Crohn's disease, 17
Crosne, 18
Cultural identity, roots and,
    viii–ix

Dandelion root, 42
Dates, in Beet-Date Ketchup,
    115

Dementia, 2–3, 5, 6. *See also*
    Cognitive decline, stopping
Desserts, 145–159
    about: coconut sugar tips, 146
    Baked Cinnamon Jicama, 154
    Beet Cake, 145–146
    Beet Panna Cotta, 154–155,
    159
    Carrot Cake Pudding, 155
    Carrot Pie, 151
    Chocolate-Beet-Coconut
    Pudding, 156
    Coconut Cream Frosting, 150
    Gluten-Free Spiced Parsnip
    Cupcakes, 147
    Healthier Carrot Cake, *144*,
    148
    Juice Pop Blueprint, 157
    Nutty Sweet Potato Ice
    Cream, 158
    Parsnip Snack Cake, 149
    Parsnip Tart, 152
    Purple Sweet Potato Pie with
    Coconut Almond Crust,
    153
    Root Juice Gelato, 158
    Rutabaga Bars, 150
    Sweet Potato Indian Pudding,
    156–157
    Whipped Coconut Topping,
    151
Diabetes, 15, 28, 33–34, 171
Dinner. *See also* Salads, dinner;
    Soups and stews, dinner
    Barley Bake, 131
    Braised Brisket and Roots,
    140–141
    Carrot-Hazelnut Puree, 135
    Millet-Root Pilaf, 132
    Moroccan Quinoa with
    Roots, 133
    Roast Chicken and Root
    Vegetables with Mustard-
    Rosemary Sauce, 139
    Roasted Root Vegetables, 136
    Root Vegetable Curry, 141
    Salmon on a Bed of Rooty
    Lentils, 142
    Sauté of Root Vegetables, 137
    Smashed Purple Potatoes,
    134
    Turkish Celeriac, 138
    Vegan Shepherd's Pie,
    142–143
Dips. *See* Condiments and
    sauces
Drinks, 41–49
    Beet-and-Celeriac-Greens
    Smoothie, 43

Beetroot Latte, 41
Burdock Tea, 42
Carrot-Mango Lassi, 45
Carrot-Orange Juice, 49
Celeriac Juice, 48
Homemade Burdock and
    Dandelion Soda, 42
Parsnip Smoothie, 45
PPL Juice, 48
Radish Jicama Juice, 47
Red Smoothie, *40*, 46
Rutabaga Juice Cocktail, 47
Salsify Tea, 43
Sweet Potato Smoothie, 46
Veggie Fusion Juice, 49

Eggs, in breakfast dishes, 61,
    65, 66
Exfoliating mask, 163

Facial care. *See* Beauty recipes
Family, tradition and roots, ix
Fatty liver disease, 33–34
Fennel, 32
Fertility, cassava and, 13
Fiber, 2, **4**, 8, 10, 12, 15, 17, 20,
    22, 25, 28, 30, 33, 34–35, 37
Fish and seafood
    Grilled Tuna, Turnip, and
        Radish Salad, 124–125
    Parsnip Salmon Pancakes,
        58
    Salmon and Roasted Root
        Veggie Salad, 91–92
    Salmon on a Bed of Rooty
        Lentils, 142
    Salmon-Veggie Chowder,
        129
    Spicy Fish Taco Bowls, 88
    Superfood Salmon Bowl, 86
    Tropical Shrimp Salad with
        Roots, *122*, 126
    Turnip Snack, 102
Fluoride, **5**, 25
Folate (vitamin B9), 2, **5**, 8, 12,
    20, 22, 25, 28, 30, 37
Freezing roots, 170
Fries recipes, 80–81
Frittata, cabbage-carrot with
    rosemary, 61

Garlic, as bulb, 32
Glaucoma, 11
Greens
    about: edibility of, 168–169;
        precautions, 44, 168–169;
        root greens and their uses,
        44, 168
    Barley-Root Soup, 127

Beet-and-Celeriac-Greens
    Smoothie, 43
Fresh Green Sauce, 113
Growing roots, 169. *See also*
    specific roots

Hair care. *See* Beauty recipes
Ham. *See* Pork
Hash, 62, 63, 66
Health benefits. *See specific roots*
Heart health/cardiovascular
    disease, 3, 6, 11, 170
History of roots. *See specific roots*
Horseradish, 18, 27
Hummus, 120–121
Hypertension. *See* Blood pressure

Immune system, strengthening,
    4, 5, 7, 23, 32
Inflammation, reducing, 8, 12,
    23, 26, 30–31
Intestinal disorders/infections,
    17, 34
Iron, x, **6**, 22, 33, 35

Jicama, 17–19
    about: botanical background,
        19; buying, 17; general
        information, 17–19; greens
        and their uses, 44; growing
        information, 19; health-
        supporting role, 17; history
        of, 19; nutrition profile, 17;
        storing, 17–19; things to
        be aware of, 19; using/uses,
        x, 19, 44
    Baked Cinnamon Jicama, 154
    Collard Root Wrap, 83
    Jicama Brightener, 164
    Jicama, Radish, and Pepita
        Salad, 90
    Mexicali Jicama Sticks, 100
    Radish Jicama Juice, 47
    Radish-Jicama Salsa, 112
    Roasted Root Vegetables with
        Ham, 64
    Rooty Pinwheels, 101
    Shredded Root Salad
        Blueprint, 92–93
    Southwestern Salad, 125–126
    Spicy Fish Taco Bowls, 88
    Spinach Root Salad, 93
    Superfood Salmon Bowl, 86
    Tropical Shrimp Salad with
        Roots, *122*, 126
Juice Pop Blueprint, 157
Juices
    Carrot-Orange Juice, 49
    Celeriac Juice, 48

PPL Juice, 48
Radish Jicama Juice, 47
Root Juice Gelato, 158
Rutabaga Juice Cocktail, 47
Veggie Fusion Juice, 49

Ketchup, beet-date, 115
Kohlrabi, 32

Lassi, carrot-mango, *40*, 45
Latkes, turnip, 60
Leeks, as bulbs, 32
Lemons and limes. *See* Citrus
Lentils. *See* Beans and other
    legumes
Leukemia, 20, 36
Libido, enhancing, 8
Liver health, 26, 31, 33–34,
    42, 47
Lotus root, 18
Lunch, 77–97. *See also* Salads;
    Sandwiches and wraps;
    Soups, stews, and chilis
    Autumn Quinoa Bowl, 87
    Parsnip Fries, 81
    Rooty Buddha Bowl, 89
    Rutabaga Fries, *76*, 80
    Spicy Fish Taco Bowls, 88
    Superfood Salmon Bowl, 86
Lutein, **6**, 10, 15, 22, 25
Lycopene, **6**, 10

Macrobiotics, ix, 89
Magnesium, **6**, 8, 20, 22, 30,
    33, 35
Manganese, 2, **6**, 8, 10, 15, 20,
    22, 28, 30, 35, 37
Mangoes, *40*, 45, *122*, 126
Masks, 163
Memory, dementia and, 2–3,
    5, 6
Metric conversions, 171, 173
Millet-Root Pilaf, 132
Muffins. *See* Breakfast
Mushrooms, 67–68, 142–143
Mustard, sweet potato, 116

Niacin (vitamin B3), **6**, 12, 22,
    33, 35
Nutrients in roots, 4–7. *See also*
    specific nutrients
Nutrition profiles. *See specific*
    roots
Nuts and seeds
    Autumn Quinoa Bowl, 87
    Barley Bake, 131
    Carrot Cake Muffins, *50*, 52
    Carrot-Hazelnut Puree, 135
    Glory Muffins, 53

GORP Carrot Chips, 99
Grain-Free Porridge, 73
Hearty Carrot Juice Pulp
    Crackers, 104
Jicama, Radish, and Pepita
    Salad, 90
Nutty Sweet Potato Ice
    Cream, 158
Roasted Sweet Potato Salad
    with Chipotle Vinaigrette,
    90–91
Spinach Root Salad, 93
Superfood Skordalia, 119
Sweet Potato–Peanut Stew,
    97
Sweet Root Chia Pudding, 75
Warm Root Salad, 70

Oats
    about: colorful, cooking in
        beet/carrot juice, 73; types/
        forms of, 74
    Autumn Spice Oatmeal, 71
    Carrot Cake Oatmeal, 72–73
    Oatmeal-Beet Exfoliating
        mask, 163
    Rooty Rolled Oat Risotto,
        67–68
Oca, 18
Omega-3 fatty acids, 2, **6**, 8, 10,
    12, 17, 20, 22, 24, 25, 28,
    30, 35, 37
Onions, as bulbs, 32
Oranges. *See* Citrus
Osteoporosis, 15
Oxidative damage, in vitro, 37
Oxidative stress, combatting,
    8, 20

Pain, reducing, 30–31
Panna cotta, beet, 154–155, *159*
Parsley root, 18
Parsnips, 20–21
    about: botanical background,
        21; buying, 20; general
        information, 20–21; greens
        precaution, 44, 168–169;
        growing information, 21;
        health-supporting role, 20;
        history of, 21; nutrition
        profile, 20; storing, 20;
        things to be aware of, 21;
        using/uses, x, 20–21
    Baked Root Chips, *98*,
        102–103
    Barley-Root Soup, 127
    Beef-and-Root Stew, 128
    Braised Brisket and Roots,
        140–141

Classy Hash, 63
Glory Muffins, 53
Gluten-Free Spiced Parsnip Cupcakes, 147
Grain-Free Porridge, 73
Hearty Carrot Juice Pulp Crackers, 104
Moroccan Quinoa with Roots, 133
Parsnip-Carrot Pickle, 108
Parsnip Fries, 81
Parsnip Griddle Cakes, 57
Parsnip Salmon Pancakes, 58
Parsnip Smoothie, 45
Parsnip Snack Cake, 149
Parsnip Tart, 152
PPL Juice, 48
Roasted Root Vegetables, 136
Roasted Root Vegetables with Ham, 64
Root Vegetable Curry, 141
Root Veggie Pita, 84
Rooty Breakfast Cake, 55
Rooty Buddha Bowl, 89
Salmon and Roasted Root Veggie Salad, 91–92
Spiced Root Dal Soup, 130
Superfood Skordalia with, 119
Sweet Root Chia Pudding, 75
Vegan Shepherd's Pie, 142–143
Veggie Thin Crackers, 105
Warm Root Salad, 70
Pears, 48
Pesto, 63
Phosphorus, 6, 15, 20, 22, 28, 30, 33, 35
Phytonutrients, about, 28, 37, 38, 170
Phytosterols, 2, 7, 25, 37
Pickles. See Condiments and sauces
Poisonous roots, 169
Pork
Celeriac Hash, 62
Roasted Root Vegetables with Ham, 64
Sweet Potato Bacon (or Not) Wrap, 85
Potassium, 2, 7, 8, 10, 15, 17, 20, 22, 25, 28, 30, 33, 35, 37
Potatoes, 22–24
about: annual consumption, vi, 24; botanical background, 23; buying, 23; chip origins, 24; consumption statistics, 169; "fancying up," x;

French fries, 24; general information, 23–25; gold, 22; greens precaution, 44, 169; growing information, 24; health-supporting role, 23; history of, 24; leftover cooked uses, 134; national days for, 24; nutrition profile by color variety, 22; pink/red-flesh, 22; popularity of, vi; purple, 22; storing, 23; things to be aware of, 25; using/uses, 23, 25, 44, 134; varieties, 24
Baked Root Chips, 98, 102–103
Carrot-Hazelnut Puree, 135
Classy Hash, 63
Cocktail Potatoes, 103
Roasted Root Vegetables, 136
Roasted Root Vegetables with Ham, 64
Root Vegetable Curry, 141
Root Veggie Pita, 84
Salmon and Roasted Root Veggie Salad, 91–92
Salmon-Veggie Chowder, 129
Shine and Body Rinse (for hair), 165
Smashed Purple Potatoes, 134
Superfood Skordalia, 119
Vegan Shepherd's Pie, 142–143
Protein, 2, 4, 7, 10, 12, 15, 17, 20, 22, 25, 28, 30, 33, 35, 36, 37

Quinoa
Autumn Quinoa Bowl, 87
Breakfast Quinoa, 71–72
Moroccan Quinoa with Roots, 133
Rooty Buddha Bowl, 89
Southwestern Salad, 125–126
Spicy Fish Taco Bowls, 88
Sweet Potato Protein Burgers, 76, 82

Radishes, 25–27
about: botanical background, 27; buying, 26; flavor origin, 27; general information, 26–27; greens and their uses, 44, 168; growing information, 27; health-supporting role, 25–26; Mexican festivals for, 27; nutrition profile, 25;

storing, 26; things to be aware of, 27; using/uses, 27, 44; varieties, 27
Cannellini Veggie Sandwich, 84
Creamy Cream-Free Radish Dip, 118
Grilled Tuna, Turnip, and Radish Salad, 124–125
Jicama, Radish, and Pepita Salad, 90
Radish Jicama Juice, 47
Radish-Jicama Salsa, 112
Radish Snack, 100
Roasted Root Vegetables with Ham, 64
Spicy Fish Taco Bowls, 88
Spinach Root Salad, 93
Superfood Salmon Bowl, 86
Tropical Shrimp Salad with Roots, 122, 126
Ramps, as bulbs, 32
Resources, 172
Rhizomes, 167
Riboflavin (vitamin B2), 7, 30, 35
Rice, 86, 88
Roots. See also specific roots
affordability, 1–2
benefits and appeal, 1–2
bulbs confused with, 32, 167
consumption limits, 171
cultural identity and, viii–ix
edibility of, 167–168
family, tradition and, ix
flavor appeal, 1
freezing, 170
greens of. See Greens
growing, 169
intrepid nature of, 1
macrobiotics and, ix, 89
memories of, vi–viii
nutrients in, 4–7. See also specific nutrients
nutritional benefits, 1
poisonous, 169
questions and answers, 167–171
raw vs. cooked, 168
rhizomes vs., 167
superfood status, 170
unusual, 18
using/uses, ix–xi
Rutabagas, 28–30
about: botanical background, 29; buying, 29; cultural identity and, viii–ix; general information, 29–30; greens and their uses, 44, 168;

growing information, 29–30; health-supporting role, 28–29; history of, 29; nutrition profile, 28; storing, 29; things to be aware of, 30; using/uses, x, 29, 30, 44
Barley-Root Soup, 127
Braised Brisket and Roots, 140–141
Classy Hash, 63
Mashed Rutabaga, 69
Mexicali Rutabaga Muffins, 54
Roast Chicken and Root Vegetables with Mustard-Rosemary Sauce, 139
Roasted Root Vegetables, 136
Roasted Root Vegetables with Ham, 64
Root Veggie Pita, 84
Rutabaga Bars, 150
Rutabaga Fries, 76, 80
Rutabaga Juice Cocktail, 47
Salmon and Roasted Root Veggie Salad, 91–92
Sauté of Root Vegetables, 137
Superfood Caponata, 114

Salads
Brunch Salad, 67
Celeriac Salad, 69
Grated Carrot Salad, 69
Jicama, Radish, and Pepita Salad, 90
Roasted Sweet Potato Salad with Chipotle Vinaigrette, 90–91
Salmon and Roasted Root Veggie Salad, 91–92
Shredded Root Salad Blueprint, 92–93
Spinach Root Salad, 93
Warm Root Salad, 70
Salads, dinner, 123–126
Celeriac Lentil Salad, 123–124
Grilled Tuna, Turnip, and Radish Salad, 124–125
Southwestern Salad, 125–126
Tropical Shrimp Salad with Roots, 122, 126
Salsify and scorzonera, 30–33
about: botanical background, 31; buying, 31; general information, 31–33; greens and their uses, 44, 168;

growing information, 33; health-supporting role, 30–31; history of, 33; nutrition profile, 30; storing, 31; things to be aware of, 33; using/uses, 31, 33, 44
Barley Bake, 131
Braised Brisket and Roots, 140–141
Burdock or Salsify Relish, 110–111
Rooty Buddha Bowl, 89
Salsify Tea, 43
Simple Cream of Salsify Soup, 97
Sandwiches and wraps, 77–85
Beef-Root Burgers, 77–78
Beet Bean Burgers, 78
Cannellini Veggie Sandwich, 84
Carrot Falafel Balls, 79
Collard Root Wrap, 83
Root Veggie Pita, 84
Sweet Potato and Black Bean Breakfast Wraps, 65
Sweet Potato Bacon (or Not) Wrap, 85
Sweet Potato Protein Burgers, 76, 82
Saponins, 13
Sauces. See Condiments and sauces
Scorzonera. See Salsify and scorzonera
Seeds. See Nuts and seeds
Selenium, 7
Sex drive, enhancing, 8
Shallots, as bulbs, 32
Shepherd's pie, vegan, 142–143
Sides, breakfast, 67–70
Sides, starchy, 131–134
Sides, veggie, 135–138
Smoothies/blender drinks, 43–46
Beet-and-Celeriac-Greens Smoothie, 43
Carrot-Mango Lassi, 40, 45
Parsnip Smoothie, 45
Red Smoothie, 40, 46
Sweet Potato Smoothie, 46
Snacks, 99–105. See also Condiments and sauces
about: ideas for grated roots, 100; veggie dippers, 114
Baked Root Chips, 98, 102–103
Cocktail Potatoes, 103
GORP Carrot Chips, 99

Hearty Carrot Juice Pulp Crackers, 104
Mexicali Jicama Sticks, 100
Radish Snack, 100
Rooty Pinwheels, 101
Turnip Snack, 102
Veggie Thin Crackers, 105
Soups and stews, dinner, 127–130
Barley-Root Soup, 127
Beef-and-Root Stew, 128
Salmon-Veggie Chowder, 129
Spiced Root Dal Soup, 130
Soups, stews, and chilis, 93–97
Beet-Bean Chili, 93–94
Carrot-Burdock Bisque, 94–95
Easy Root Soup Blueprint, 95–96
Simple Cream of Salsify Soup, 97
Sweet Potato–Peanut Stew, 97
Spinach
Spinach Root Salad, 93
Veggie Fusion Juice, 49
Spreads. See Condiments and sauces
Stamina, improving, 2
Storing roots. See specific roots
Stroke, reducing risk, 12–13
Sugar, coconut, 146
Sunchokes, 33–35
about: artichokes and, ix; botanical background, 34; buying, 34; general information, 34–35; greens and their uses, 44; growing information, 34; health-supporting role, 33–34; history of, 34; nutrition profile, 33; things to be aware of, 34–35; using/uses, 34, 35, 44
Roasted Root Vegetables, 136
Roasted Root Vegetables with Ham, 64
Roasted Sunchokes, 69
Root Veggie Pita, 84
Sunchoke Pickles, 109–110
Sweet potatoes, 35–37
about: botanical background, 36; buying, 36; general information, 36–37; greens and their uses, 44, 168; growing information, 37; health-supporting role, 36;

history of, 36–37; nutrition profile, 35; storing, 36; using/uses, 36, 37, 44
Autumn Spice Oatmeal, 71
Baked Root Chips, 98, 102–103
Barley Bake, 131
Cannellini Beet Dip, 117
Celeriac Hash, 62
Grain-Free Porridge, 73
Hearty Carrot Juice Pulp Crackers, 104
Nutty Sweet Potato Ice Cream, 158
Purple Sweet Potato Pie with Coconut Almond Crust, 153
Roasted Sweet Potato Salad with Chipotle Vinaigrette, 90–91
Root Vegetable Curry, 141
Rooty Rolled Oat Risotto, 67–68
Salmon and Roasted Root Veggie Salad, 91–92
Spiced Root Dal Soup, 130
Sweet Potato and Black Bean Breakfast Wraps, 65
Sweet Potato Bacon (or Not) Wrap, 85
Sweet Potato Hash with Eggs, 66
Sweet Potato Hummus, 120–121
Sweet Potato Indian Pudding, 156–157
Sweet Potato Mustard, 116
Sweet Potato–Peanut Stew, 97
Sweet Potato Protein Burgers, 76, 82
Sweet Potato Smoothie, 46
Sweet Root Chia Pudding, 75
Veggie Thin Crackers, 105
Warm Root Salad, 70

Tapioca body wash, 161
Tapioca, breakfast, 72
Taro, 18
Thiamine (vitamin B1), 7
Tiger nut, 18
Triglycerides, lowering, 17
Turnips, 37–39
about: botanical background, 39; buying, 38; general information, 38–39; greens and their uses, 44, 168; growing information, 39;

health-supporting role, 37–38; nutrition profile, 37; storing, 38; things to be aware of, 39; using/uses, 39, 44
Barley-Root Soup, 127
Beef-and-Root Stew, 128
Beef-Root Burgers, 77–78
Grilled Tuna, Turnip, and Radish Salad, 124–125
Hearty Carrot Juice Pulp Crackers, 104
Pickled Turnips, 109
Roast Chicken and Root Vegetables with Mustard-Rosemary Sauce, 139
Roasted Root Vegetables with Ham, 64
Root Vegetable Curry, 141
Rooty Buddha Bowl, 89
Rooty Pinwheels, 101
Salmon on a Bed of Rooty Lentils, 142
Superfood Salmon Bowl, 86
Superfood Skordalia with, 119
Turnip Latkes, 60
Turnip Snack, 102
Veggie Fusion Juice, 49
Veggie Thin Crackers, 105

Vegan Shepherd's Pie, 142–143
Vitamin A, 4, 10, 22, 35
Vitamin B1. See Thiamine
Vitamin B2. See Riboflavin
Vitamin B3. See Niacin
Vitamin B6, 4, 8, 10, 15, 22, 28, 30, 33, 35, 37
Vitamin B9. See Folate
Vitamin C, 2, 4, 8, 10, 12–13, 15, 17, 20, 22, 25, 28, 30, 33, 35, 37
Vitamin E, 5, 10, 15, 20, 22, 35
Vitamin K, 5

Waffles, 56, 59
Weight loss and maintenance, 8
Wounds, healing, 4, 7, 31

Yacon, 18

Zinc, 7